Praise for

WHERE THE LIGHT GETS IN

"Kimberly Williams-Paisley has written a book that is both heartbreaking and essential. I loved it for all the love it contained but also for the wealth of practical information. The Williams family went down a hard road with dementia, and we can all benefit from their experience."

—ANN PATCHETT, *NEW YORK TIMES* BESTSELLING
AUTHOR OF *BEL CANTO* AND *STATE OF WONDER*

"The relationship between a mother and daughter is one of the most complicated and meaningful there is. Kimberly Williams-Paisley writes about her own with grace, truth, and beauty as she shares her journey back to her mother in the wake of a devastating illness."

—BROOKE SHIELDS, *NEW YORK TIMES* BESTSELLING
AUTHOR OF *THERE WAS A LITTLE GIRL*

"Kim's story really resonated with me, as it will with countless others. Her beautiful, heartfelt book is an absolute must-read for mothers, daughters, and anyone dealing with a loved one living with dementia. It will also help to bring comfort to families facing any type of life-altering situation."

—ROBIN ROBERTS, *GOOD MORNING AMERICA*

"*Where the Light Gets In* is simply wonderful ... and sad ... and brave. This book will bring comfort to families who are experiencing the complex and confusing journey of progressive dementia while still celebrating moments of true joy. Williams-Paisley's narrative and the resource section will help people know they are not alone."

—ANGELA TIMASHENKA GEIGER, CHIEF STRATEGY
OFFICER, ALZHEIMER'S ASSOCIATION

"*Where the Light Gets In* left an indelible mark on my heart. The story of love and acceptance and the unbreakable bond of family, this book will be a comfort to so many families who are going through what Kim's went through and will be a much-needed source of strength for all those who read it."

—SHERYL CROW, MUSICIAN

"Generous, human, and healing; that's what this book is. Kimberly Williams-Paisley has invited us into her life and her family so that we may know ourselves better. By sharing her story with such vulnerability and honesty, she makes it accessible to everyone, with or without a personal connection to dementia. Through it, I had the experience of seeing my own family differently, understanding my desire to love more, and connecting deeply to my own stories of illness, grief, compassion, empathy, and redemption."

—CONNIE BRITTON, ACTRESS

"Informative, relatable, and heartbreaking, *Where the Light Gets In* is a must-read for those who have a loved one struggling with dementia."

—SETH MEYERS, HOST OF *LATE NIGHT WITH SETH MEYERS*

"Kimberly Williams-Paisley's experience with her mother's dementia is very moving, and you'll be touched by so much in this book. This topic needs national attention, and *Where the Light Gets In* helps bring focus to that need."

—WILLIAM SHATNER, ACTOR

WHERE THE LIGHT GETS IN

LOSING MY MOTHER only to FIND HER AGAIN

Kimberly Williams-Paisley

Foreword by Michael J. Fox

CROWN
ARCHETYPE
NEW YORK

Copyright © 2016 by Kimberly Williams-Paisley

Foreword copyright © 2016 by Michael J. Fox

All rights reserved.
Published in the United States by Crown Archetype,
an imprint of the Crown Publishing Group,
a division of Penguin Random House LLC, New York.
www.crownpublishing.com

Crown Archetype and colophon is a registered
trademark of Penguin Random House LLC.

Credits can be found on page 259, which is an extension of the copyright page.

A portion of the author's proceeds has been donated to the Alzheimer's Association.

Library of Congress Cataloging-in-Publication Data
Names: Williams-Paisley, Kimberly, 1971– author.
Title: Where the light gets in : losing my mother only to find her again / Kimberly Williams-Paisley.
Description : First edition. | New York : Crown Archetype, [2016]
Identifiers: LCCN 2015036024 | ISBN 9781101902950 (hardback) | ISBN 9781101902974 (tradepaper) | ISBN 9781101902967 (ebook)
Subjects: LCSH: Williams-Paisley, Kimberly, 1971– | Aphasic persons–Biography. | Mothers and daughters–Biography. | Dementia–Patients–Family relationships. | BISAC: BIOGRAPHY & AUTOBIOGRAPHY / Personal Memoirs. | HEALTH & FITNESS / Diseases / Alzheimer's & Dementia. | BIOGRAPHY & AUTOBIOGRAPHY / Entertainment & Performing Arts.
Classification: LCC RC425 .W55 2016 | DDC 616.8/30092–dc23 LC record available at http://lccn.loc.gov/2015036024

ISBN 978-1-101-90295-0
eBook ISBN 978-1-101-90296-7

PRINTED IN THE UNITED STATES OF AMERICA

Book design by Anna Thompson
Jacket photographs: (front) Lara Porzak; (back: paper clip) Ben Enos

10 9 8 7 6 5 4 3 2 1

First Edition

For my mom

D isease, by definition, alights on an individual. But the
ripple effects of a diagnosis go far beyond a single life.
Not just patients but families, too, become accustomed to
frustration and fear as constant companions in the early
days. Fantasies of escape take hold, as does the hope against
hope that a mistake has been made. Even when some form
of acceptance is gained, it's tempting to take a diagnosis as
confirmation of our darkest views of the world: proof that
happiness is not to be trusted, that demise is the cosmic
price we have to pay for living.

And yet, as I can attest from my own experience, when
a family operates as a loving unit, it is capable of transmog-
rifying even the bleakest and most unwelcome of events.
I don't pretend to know how it works; there's a magic to
it. When the road is challenging, navigating the ups and

downs together reveals abilities we never knew we had, and the strength to carry a weight we never expected. We flex new muscles and are surprised to discover they were there all along.

Linda Williams was one of those people who come into your life—friends, family members, sometimes colleagues— whose compassion for others and outlook on life resonate with you forever. As our foundation's first major-gifts fund-raiser, she inspired our staff with her ability to convey to supporters both the complex neuroscience we were driving and the simple optimism that our efforts would speed a cure. And so, though our staff works every day with patients and families battling a progressive neurological disease, we were devastated when she revealed to us that she'd been diagnosed with a rare form of dementia, one that would diminish and then take away altogether her astounding powers of communication.

But Linda's husband, Gurney, and their grown children saw her diagnosis as a call to arms, and the support system they created was remarkable. They surrounded her with compassion, providing help when needed and making light of symptoms when they could. When Kim first wrote publicly about Linda's illness in a magazine essay, I was reminded of all the good that can come from sharing our stories, in spite of how risky it feels (something my wife, Tracy Pollan, and I remember all too well from our own experience letting the genie out of the bottle).

That magazine essay became the seed of this book,

which I'm so grateful to Kim for sharing, in all its honesty, poignancy, and humor. She has helped to rekindle a national dialogue on family, sickness, and health, and she's given countless individuals an opportunity to talk about their own experiences, struggles and fears, hopes for the future. All at a time when scientists and researchers believe we are closer than ever to breakthroughs and possible cures for the brain diseases that touch three in five American families.

Kim clearly inherited her mother's deftness with words, the same facility that used to blow everyone at our foundation away. Yet in spite of the beauty of her writing, Kim's story ultimately is one of inventing a new language, one that allows her and her mother to wordlessly convey: *I get you. You understand me. We love each other.*

Come to find out—that's enough.

Michael J. Fox

If the brain were so simple we could understand it,
we would be so simple we couldn't.

—LYALL WATSON

t was almost a picture-perfect wedding. Not the Hollywood version most people saw in *Father of the Bride*, which actually took weeks to shoot. I mean the real one. The one that took about an hour, and began a marriage that has thrived for more than thirteen years and counting.

The film was about a high-ticket formal affair. The real thing was modest by comparison. It was designed around a secret. Only our families, our officiants, and Brad's best friend, Kelley, knew we were actually getting married that day. We wanted it to be a surprise. That was our way of mixing things up a bit, of taking the pressure off the event. For years audiences had seen me as the bride from their favorite wedding movie, and I was worried people at my real ceremony would say, "It was nice, but the movie was better." And Brad, a musician, grew up playing at other people's weddings, and hated the tension he felt at every one. We were determined to make ours fun.

The only real concern I had that day was my mother, Linda. When I look back now, the pieces of the puzzle fit together in a way that they couldn't have then. My big day gave me the first glimpse into what was coming.

In the Hollywood version, Mom was just an extra, on-screen for a few seconds. You can see her there still, in the reception scene. She's wearing a sparkly gold top and giant pearl earrings–borrowed from wardrobe–and her hair is in tightly permed curls. She's laughing with Diane Keaton and drinking fake champagne. You can't hear their words, but she and Diane were giggling about pet dogs. She looks happy and self-confident.

But in the oceanside hotel room in Malibu on the day of my real wedding, Mom was crying because she wasn't part of the ceremony. She'd always loved the bustle and laughter of a party or celebration, didn't want to miss a minute of fun, and was often the last to leave. Now, it seemed, she'd only just realized that she had no role to play, no words to say, in a major family event. She felt left out.

Long before that day, Brad and I briefly discussed the simple program with my parents over the phone. We invited my dad to stand up, introduce me to Brad's guests, and talk about our family. We designed the rest of the ceremony without their input. We asked Kelley to honor his and Brad's long friendship with a little speech. We asked Brad's Baptist preacher, Mike Glenn, and my Episcopal priest, Susan Harriss, to fly out to California and marry us together. That was it. Simple and easy.

I wanted Mom to be involved in other aspects of the preparation. I sought her help on one of my dress fittings, and consulted with her on the guest list. She added more than two dozen people because she didn't want anyone to feel excluded.

Now, as we went over the specific plan hours before the ceremony, she wept. I felt terrible that she was upset about it, but I didn't know what we could add at this point. Susan stepped in and suggested that Mom read the letter of Paul to the Colossians. My mother is the least religious person in our family, and I don't know if she'd ever recited a Bible passage aloud. But she seemed comforted for the moment.

That rainy evening in the chapel at Pepperdine University, all our guests inside believed they were attending the rehearsal. They thought it strange, I'm sure—and maybe even a little annoying—that they were even asked to come. There were no ushers. No quiet organ music. No buzz of anticipation. No separation of bride's guests and groom's guests. Friends and family in casual clothes sat or wandered around as they wished. Waiting for me to arrive, my husband-to-be chatted and chewed gum.

I was back in the hotel room with my brother, Jay, and sister, Ashley, getting ready to go. Both of my siblings had lived with me at different times years before in my tiny house in Santa Monica. Jay was my housemate while he worked long hours as a camera assistant on television shows and then after he quit to become a firefighter. He slept in my second bedroom, stored his unicycle and surfboard in my basement, and helped keep a tidy home. We sometimes took meandering adventure walks to unplanned places, often winding up at the pier fifteen minutes away and riding the Ferris wheel with the last dollar bills in our pockets.

Ash crashed in my basement after she graduated from college and got cast almost immediately as the female lead in an NBC series, *Good Morning, Miami.* She was thrust into the spotlight, for better or worse, as I had been. In the hotel room, Ash had taken off her underwear and given it to me because mine was showing lines under the thin white fabric of my wedding dress—my something borrowed. I could share pretty much anything with either of my siblings, and I was grateful they were there to calm me.

We left on time. My father, Gurney, drove cautiously on the wet roads. Mom started singing Christmas songs, off-key, and Ash and Jay somewhat reluctantly joined in. It was March. They suddenly seemed manic, in serious need of stress release. "Christmas is coming, the goose is getting fat!" they screamed.

Ash and I clutched hands in the backseat, as we had before in scary times. I would be the first of the three of us to be at the altar, and we didn't know what to expect. I looked out the window at the clouds and tried to remember to take deep breaths.

We pulled up to the chapel, ducked through the rain, and ran inside. I carried a garish bouquet of multicolored my only bridesmaid, sharing my urge to reach out to our mother and help. Before either of us could, she tried again.

"If anyone has a complaint against another, forgive one another, and if anyone has . . ." She faltered. "If anyone has a complaint against another," she mumbled. "In each other." She threw her hand out to her side as though the reading were riddled with typos. When finally she finished, I realized I'd been holding my breath.

Our pale blue station wagon fishtailed down a hill on icy snow. Home was just ahead, a sharp and narrow right turn through stone pillars off Howe Place in Bronxville, New York. We were in trouble—moving faster, skidding nearly out of control. If Mom spun the wheel too hard and we missed the driveway, the Buick would whirl a hundred feet to the bottom of the street and plunge down a flight of stairs on the other side of an intersection.

There were no rules in 1979 about kids sitting in the backseat. So I was Mom's co-pilot in the front. I could feel her panic rise. I looked out the window at the cold black sky and prayed in fear to the brightest star. In my eight-year-old's world, it was the soul of my grandfather, who was something of a saint to me and had died months earlier.

Grandpa, I prayed. *Save us. We need you.*

"Shit," Mom said. I'd never heard her say that word. I prayed harder. *Grandpa, PLEASE. Help Mom.*

We were entering the perilous turn. She seemed more alarmed than I'd ever seen her as her hands gripped the wheel. I struggled to keep my eye on that star. Time slowed. My mother screamed.

"Shit! Shit! Shit in a bucket!"

The car swerved, turned, and slid between the pillars. A layer of snow on our driveway crunched under the tires, and then we were in our garage, safe.

There was a silence, broken a few moments later by tentative laughter.

"*What* about a bucket?" I snickered.

"Sorry," Mom said, a little embarrassed. "That was just something your grandfather used to say."

A miracle. I thanked the star.

For one of the first times in my life, my mom had become someone else right before my eyes. I was both startled and intrigued. Who was this mother of mine?

I'VE ASKED MYSELF THAT QUESTION many times since she was diagnosed with primary progressive aphasia, a rare form of dementia, in 2005 at the age of sixty-two. She has since become someone I barely recognize.

I miss her—the mom from long ago, before any of this started.

As I write this, I'm looking at two black-and-white photos taken on my wedding day more than thirteen years ago. The separate shots of Mom and me are nestled artfully together under clear, clean glass and a bright white beveled mat.

After Brad had kissed me, a gospel choir scattered secretly throughout the congregation stood up and belted out "Oh Happy Day." Brad and I paraded back up the aisle and then snuck into a balcony to watch our dressed-down, rowdy guests. They were cheering, waving, singing "Amazing Grace" and a raucous "Praise God."

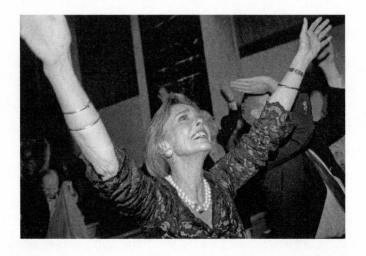

And there was Mom in the middle of everyone. She seemed euphoric.

Later I arranged the two separate photos of that moment in the same black frame. She is in the lower corner, with her arms held high and rigid. Her one visible eye conveys a mixture of ecstasy and perhaps fear about what was beginning to happen to her. Above her picture is one of me. I'm looking up, laughing. I am lifted by the love of my family, especially my mother.

Below the photos is a quote from something I'd told an interviewer at a magazine a few years earlier for their Mother's Day issue. I copied it down in black ink: *She's still that voice in my head that says, "Go for it! You can do it! Even if things are scary or difficult or you've never done them before, do them anyway!"*

I put this collage together for Mom after my wedding as a sort of peace offering. Her bouts of anger had become more frequent recently, and I was hoping to put all of the strains of the engagement and wedding behind us. I think I knew she needed encouragement. And I wanted her to know I was grateful for all that she'd given me up to that point in my life. It was true: my mother had always urged my brother and sister and me to "go for it," beginning in my earliest years.

When I was a child, we often went to Cape Cod in September to visit my grandmother after Grandpa died. Most beachgoers were content to sit on their towels at the end of the tourist season. But Mom wouldn't stand for that.

Despite the first cool whisperings of winter in the breeze or a cloudy sky, she would gather Jay, Ash, and me up off the sand at Old Silver Beach, and we'd hold hands and charge toward the water, past the lounging local residents.

"Run right into the waves!" she'd instruct. "It'll be great!"

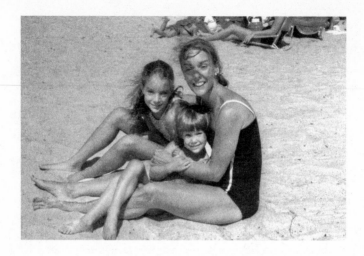

Mom knew that if we waded in tentatively, we would never get wet above the knees.

I was the oldest, the parent pleaser and rule follower. Back then, it was up to me to set a good example for Jay, three years my junior, and Ash, the youngest of the family. Mom's enthusiasm was an invitation we couldn't reject.

"We'll do it together!" she would yell. With goose bumps on our tanned skin, we raced, shrieking, into the frothy waters of Buzzards Bay, let go of one another as we fell into the waves, and bobbed back up. She was right. It *was* great.

My mother was teaching us not to shy away in the face of a challenge. Not to shrink from what was uncomfortable.

ONE DAY IN THE FUTURE, when scientists study her donated brain, they'll find signs of her disease. They might see plaque—waste material that looks like dust balls under the microscope. They may zoom inside the cells, searching for tangles resembling a jumble of spaghetti. Her brain overall will most certainly be smaller than normal, and some of the tissue might be slightly yellow or green instead of the usual gray.

But they won't be able to detect my mother's courage. They won't see her stubbornness, or humor, or infectious passion for life. They won't be able to measure how much she loved her family or what kind of parent she was.

My mother is not her disease.

She was the one who got me to appreciate the excitement of thunderstorms. When hurricanes threatened, while many residents were nailing plywood over their windows, Mom was driving us to the beach to see the wild wind churn the waves. It was her voice in my head that told me to go to the cattle-call audition for *Father of the Bride* when part of me wanted to stay in my safe dorm room. Hers was the whisper in my heart that urged me to say yes to the adventure of flying upside down in a biplane in the middle of Africa when I was twenty-four.

Seek out adventures, she told us. *Come back with stories.*

In the meantime, she didn't tolerate whining. It wasn't in her genetic makeup. Her British grandfather survived four and a half years in a Japanese prison camp in Hong Kong but didn't talk about it after he came home. Her stockbroker father, George Payne, never outwardly despaired when markets plummeted. "It's only money," he would say.

Once I saw my grandmother Betty pull a dish out of a hot oven with her bare hands, and she didn't even flinch. My mother's family history was a tale of determination and endurance, and it influenced the way she raised us—including the way she reacted when anyone in the family got sick. When I was about ten, Mom gave me an eye roll when she overheard me on the phone with my father describing in detail the way the cut on my right palm felt after I'd fallen and gashed it on a rock.

"Pain, sharp pain, pain, sharp pain," I said, milking the attention.

"Oh, brother," Mom said. "You're fine." *No big deal. Get back out there.* It healed, and she was right. I was fine, even though I still have quite a scar.

Mom launched me at an early age toward escapades and quests, some braver than she'd ever attempted. And her deep, no-nonsense love helped keep my feet rooted to the ground.

But as Mom's illness began to overtake her, dementia distorted her view of the world and erupted as extreme sadness, rage, and fear. Gradually I lost sight of the mother I used to know. I was shocked by the woman who seemed more and more alien.

My family made many missteps. I regret the things I didn't have the nerve to discuss out loud. I wish I hadn't listened to Mom's misguided requests for secrecy and autonomy rather than to rational, practical advice from people outside the family who could have offered help to both of my parents. I'm sad that I didn't keep a closer watch on my father, my mother's primary caregiver. I'm sorry I had to be a long-distance caregiver, caught between tending my mom and mothering my own children. I hate that my sister wound up carrying so much of the burden.

Eventually, though, surprising blessings began to emerge. As I begin this story of my mother, I realize that our lives today are no longer black and white. I see Mom and me in a different frame now. I believe we're healed in ways we couldn't have foreseen.

THE WOMAN I VISIT TODAY can no longer act as a mother or wife. Her single room and bath in her new home is on the fifth and highest floor, the last stop for residents requiring advanced "memory care." She sits in a wheelchair much of the time and rarely speaks. Her head droops to the right. Her expression is vacant. She sleeps often.

But her caregivers love her. They say she is impish. And empathetic—she senses whether the people around her are happy or having a hard day. She makes a face if someone is being inappropriate, and she often laughs at the sound of music. She occasionally still seems to know some things. I continue to learn from her, in profound ways.

Today she's near the counter where nurse assistants dish out a hot lunch. Her wheelchair faces a bank of curtainless windows with a panoramic view of lush tree-tops. I don't know how much of her own story, or mine, she remembers now.

She sucks Fresca or cranberry juice mixed with water through a straw when I put it to her lips. I offer her minestrone soup, and she clamps down on the spoon and won't let it go. I wait. She releases and sighs, closing her eyes.

I wipe a smear of soup off her chin with a napkin. Her eyes open and look at me. *Connection!* She shakes her tilted head slightly.

"Why?" she asks. It is a question she has asked before. It is one I ask a lot. *Why? Why is this happening to you, Mom?*

I imagine what she's thinking. *Why can't I have an apple martini? Why are you staring at me? Why am I in this place with all these strange people?*

"I don't know," I answer, and wait. She sighs.

"Shit," she says.

"Shit in a bucket," I answer. And she laughs, mouth open wide and eyes sparkling. For an instant there she is again.

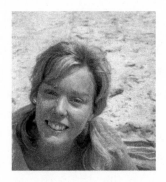

don't know if Linda Payne Williams ever thought she'd be a mother. The year I was conceived, my parents were living out their dreams as foreign correspondents. They had quit solid jobs with steady pay at *Newsday*, given up a new apartment near a beach in suburban Long Island, and said goodbye to family and friends in New York. Now, in 1970, they were freelance writers in a walk-up flat in London, feeding shillings into a stand-alone heater and cuddling to stay warm. Dad called my mother "Scout" because of her brave pioneer spirit. A single table was their office. They wore down the only typewriter ribbon they'd brought to England and reused sheets of paper by filling up every available blank space.

The first word about me appears on one of those pages, above my dad's handwritten notes for an article. Mom grabbed it and scribbled her breaking news in the corner as she received the results over the phone from the pregnancy test: "Positive."

Even after they knew she was expecting, they accepted an assignment from *Newsday* to write a feature story on the simmering conflict in Northern Ireland between Protestants and Catholics.

Dad went on foot patrol through dark Belfast streets alongside British troops searching deserted houses for crude bomb factories. He wore a flak jacket lent to him to protect him from explosion fragments, secretly hoping he'd have a Hemingway moment where he'd have to dive for cover or duck a bullet, all for the sake of the story. In a gesture toward more-responsible parenting, Mom—who usually would have accompanied him—reluctantly chose to stay at the hotel.

Dad survived without a scratch, and the next day they flew back to the States. It would be the last time either of my parents would take on a dangerous assignment, or even drive above the speed limit. Planned or not, raising a family soon became their center-ring adventure.

Mom delivered me three weeks early on September 14, 1971. Her water broke, and four hours later she was a mother. According to her tattered but elaborate record of my every moment, I weighed four pounds, seven and a half ounces and lived in an incubator for a day or so, until I was healthy enough to go home.

My head was hardly bigger than a tennis ball, my body the size of a kitten's. One of Mom's friends met me for the first time when my mother was cleaning up their apartment in Bronxville. She'd wrapped me in a long blanket trailing off toward the ground. The visitor was terrified that the vacuum cleaner might suck up the end of the blanket with tiny me in it.

"She's fine," Mom insisted.

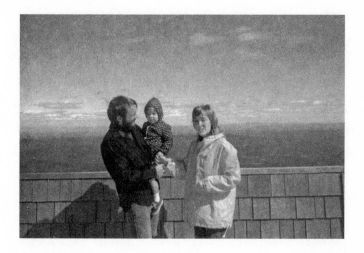

I thrived, and the family grew. Jay was born in 1974, and we moved from an apartment into a small house. Then Ashley surprised everyone in 1978. Mom and Dad bought a bigger house, and my father churned out articles from his home office, while my mother officially stopped working to take care of us.

Dad's freelance sales were barely enough to support a wife and three kids in the '70s. For years we bought groceries on sale and got our shoes two sizes too big so we could grow into them. The house became chaotic. Stacks of old newspapers, letters, and unfinished to-do lists piled up on the floors and in corners, enough to become end tables, topped off with a tissue box or an old cup of coffee.

We all tried to pitch in at home, doing dishes and laundry and trying to keep track of our pets—hamsters, fish, a parakeet, guinea pigs, mice, and a couple of snakes over the years. But my parents could take only so much of this "help" from their three small children. Sometimes my mother's stoic façade cracked, and she buckled under the strain of being a homemaker and raising her brood. I can hear her voice when she was stressed. She sounded like a crow, cawing at us to clean our rooms, tie our shoes, get in the car, and "stop fighting about who sits where!" We were often late for something.

My father's job was to stay calm and put out emotional fires or mediate between my mother and us. He convened family meetings, usually after Mom had already hit her breaking point. He gathered us at the kitchen table, where my mother sat with her arms crossed, her face red from crying.

"Nobody's very happy right now," he would say. "So let's go around the table and each talk about our needs." At the first of these sessions, I got confused. I thought, *We're going to talk about our knees?*

But the meetings usually comforted Mom, and with our apologies and promises to chip in more, she quickly recovered.

OFTEN MY PARENTS THREW SOME of the clutter into the laundry room or closets and invited people over. It was in front of these dear family friends that I first got my acting chops. I directed Jay and myself in our simple original productions—musicals, usually, meaning one or two songs and a few lines of dialogue. Following an afternoon of rehearsals, we felt confident enough to charge our parents' guests a nickel to see the show. On a good night we could make more than fifty cents. My mother supported our business acumen and taught us about money at an early age. Unlike the other moms I knew, she insisted that we pay her back for all supplies when we built a lemonade stand outside our house. There were no freebies. On the other hand, once a year Mom redefined that word. My parents splurged on a special date at a nearby clambake, an annual all-you-can-eat buffet. Without apologies, my mother took a plastic-lined purse she'd bought especially for the occasion and went through the line at least twice, first filling a plate or two for herself, and then stuffing her bag full of whole lobsters, pieces of cake, and jam-filled cookies to bring home to her delighted children.

When night came at our home and everyone had put on their pajamas and brushed their teeth, my mother relaxed and celebrated, reclining against her worn blue corduroy "throne" pillow beside a generous splash of Heaven Hill bourbon on ice in a wineglass. I rested my head on my mother's lap and she scratched my back as she read to me *The Velveteen Rabbit, Charlotte's Web,* or *A Wrinkle in Time,* acting out characters' voices and conveying all the passion of the story. She paused as she turned each page to take a sip. I can still hear the clink of the cubes and her happy sigh. And then she kept reading.

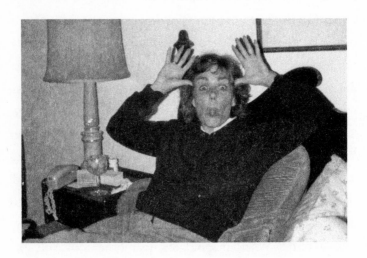

Though she felt overwhelmed at times, Mom bounced back from all of the challenging moments of my childhood with exuberance and strength. Ultimately, I think, she would have said being a mother was the most rewarding job she ever had.

. . .

IN MY EARLY TEEN YEARS, my dad got a job as senior editor at *Omni* magazine, which changed my life. Now my parents were able to scrape up enough—seven thousand dollars a year, they often reminded me—to send me to a private school in the Bronx called Fieldston, for seventh and eighth grade. The school was more than half an hour's drive from home, and most of my classmates were from Manhattan—smart, sophisticated, cultured, and scary. Mom thought I might have trouble fitting in, and so before school started she went to great lengths to befriend the mother of a classmate, Joanne. This paid off. It scored me an invite to Joanne's pool party.

No sooner had we arrived than one of the girls asked if I wanted to be a participant in their diving contest.

"Sure," I said, desperate to belong. But I hadn't thought it through. I was a good swimmer but had never learned proper diving technique. My future classmates watched as I climbed the few steps to the diving board. Mom held my towel by the side of the pool. The springy platform launched me a foot or two into the air.

For half a second I was flying. I felt great. Then I was horizontal. That is to say, not actually diving. On the way down, I saw it coming. I hit the surface in a fierce belly flop.

When I emerged from the water and saw their faces,

everyone looked horrified. Their silence stung me as much as the impact with the cruel, hard water.

"Are you all right?" one of them asked. I wasn't convinced that she cared.

"Yeah, fine." I shrugged. My cheeks were burning, my thighs throbbing. If I'd said another word, I would have sobbed. My mother wrapped a towel around me as I pulled myself out of the water.

"Wanna go put your stuff down in the dressing room?" she said brightly, as though nothing were wrong. She knew the agony I was in. She was helping me save face.

"Sure!" I said, equally cheerfully. It wasn't our style to acknowledge that something terrible had just happened.

Once we were alone together in the changing room, Mom hugged me while I cried as quietly as I could. Looking into her eyes, knowing she saw me and loved me in all of my embarrassment and awkwardness, gave me the courage to smile and head out to the party for the next round.

"It'll be a good story one day," Mom would always say at moments like this.

I can't imagine what led me to sign up for Fieldston's talent show a few months later. Just going to school was giving me hives, but for some reason I thought, *What the hell. Why don't I just do a lip sync and dance to Taco's version of "Puttin' on the Ritz"? It just feels right.* Whatever innocence I had left allowed me to ignore the possibility of disaster.

My parents told me later that the head of the school

called them and confided that she was worried I was setting myself up for failure. I was the only seventh grader who'd dared to sign up to perform. Mom and Dad spelled out the risks and asked me gently if I was—*um—sure I wanted to go ahead?* I said that I did, and from that point forward they became my cheerleaders and support team. Dad sharpened my every dance move (definitely the wrong parent for the job), including a corny pratfall. Mom helped me figure out what to wear—a black leotard, pink tights, and a top hat. She found a black cane to complete the outfit.

The night of the show, they stood at the back of the auditorium, more nervous than I was. The master of ceremonies announced that I was the youngest student to appear in the production. The audience erupted in cheers. I strode into the spotlight on the strength of that sound. I got a laugh on the fall, and I had a blast. There were no belly flops. Two and a half minutes later, I floated offstage listening to raucous applause, surely not because of my talent, but because I was the underdog and had given everything I had.

Backstage, a senior dancer, tall and kind, opened his arms and embraced me.

"Miss Cabaret!" he said. Life started looking up. I couldn't wait to perform again.

In many ways, my parents have always been at the back of the room. The support I felt from them that day gave me resolve to take the leap in front of that intimidating audience, and many others in years to come. I knew they'd be there to help me put myself back together with every subsequent failure—or at least to help me craft a good story out of it.

I felt their presence even when we weren't in the same place. When I left home the first time, years later, for a month at Phillips Exeter Academy, the summer after my sophomore year in high school, Mom wrote me a letter. We were all sad to be apart.

Dear Kim—

It's been two weeks since that first Monday morning when Daddy and I sat at breakfast, slumped. We felt like there was a big hole upstairs where you used to be. . . . Ashley has a middle ear infection from spending 8 hours a day under water. The new car is happily slurping up gasoline and Daddy put a scratch in the bumper. Jay is rolling in the dough from his paper route. He allows Ashley to come with him on collection days, with pigtails and cherub smile, to increase his tips.

But some things are still the same: Your room is still as you left it. The dining room table still has piles of paperwork. (But Grandma coming may help with all that—I'll have to clean everything up.)

Bless you—and keep up the good work. You've got a cheering squad here: a private applause section.

Loving you—
Mom

That's what my mother was for me during my childhood, more than anything else: my private applause section. And I understand now what she means about an empty space where a much-loved person used to be.

CHAPTER

3

learned to lie in my teens. It was liberating after years of striving to be a model child.

I told Mom that my boyfriend's parents would *absolutely* be at the party at his house when really they were away for the weekend. I said I'd take a taxi home. Instead, I rode shotgun a little too fast in a popular kid's dilapidated car. I fibbed when I said I'd spent an evening watching a movie with a friend when actually I was drinking beer with a crowd of kids on the local golf course. When the police arrived, I tore my shin open trying to climb over a thorn bush. Mom saw the gash. "I just tripped at Amy's house," I said. She seemed to believe me, maybe because both of us preferred to think I was a good girl.

As the oldest of three siblings, I wanted to appear flawless. It may have seemed to people who knew our family as if I could tell my mother anything, but the truth was some topics were off-limits. Mom could be a wonderfully supportive listener when she wanted to hear what I was saying—about my next English paper or a squabble with a girlfriend. But more sensitive discussions about other aspects of teen life were smothered before they began.

One day when I was about twelve, I asked her if it was okay to shave under my arms. She said, "I was wondering when you were going to notice you needed to," and that was the end of the discussion. I remember thinking, *Why didn't you just tell me?*

We never had a sit-down chat about the birds and the bees. Mom sent Dad to my room to do that. And there are some things a daughter just doesn't want to hear from her father, no matter how cool he is. Like "Your breasts will become cone-shaped."

Ew, Dad! Really?

I turned to my friends for acceptance, support, and information during those years, and worked hard not to disappoint either of my parents. But that meant I lived a partly secret life, hiding my teen rebellion and missing some of the guidance I needed from them. It was an unfortunate cycle, and Mom and I drifted apart. She worried about me, no doubt, and sensed the distance between us. Perhaps as an attempt to be more involved in my life, she offered unsolicited advice on the choices she knew about—how I spent my time (not enough on homework), who my friends were (some stayed out too late and partied too much), and what I wore (she hated my glasses and my ripped jeans). She was also having trouble sleeping, suffered from headaches, and got increasingly annoying skin rashes from the sun and allergies. I'm sure I was less forgiving than I should've been.

She is too controlling, I thought. My curfew was earlier than all of my friends'. I agreed to wake my mother up to tell her I was home safely, but that system was torturous for both of us. I tried myriad ways to do it gently—a whisper, a light touch on her arm. But every time, she bolted up in bed and shrieked.

Secretly I rolled my eyes. *Why can't she just relax?*

It was obvious when my mother was upset, not initially because she told me so, but because she started closing doors a little harder than usual, or gave me one-word answers until I begged her to say what was wrong. My family, including my more-passive father, shared a common understanding: *Nobody's happy if Mom's not.*

Though I hated her criticism, I knew she loved me. Her intentions were good. She wanted me to become a strong, self-sufficient, intelligent adult, a better person than she.

I DID FEEL HER FULL support when it came to my dream of becoming an actress. She thought the prospect was as exciting as I did, and she loved watching me perform, but she was never a typical stage mom. Auditioning should be fun, she told me, and if it wasn't, I shouldn't do it. Her faith that my goal might be realistic helped both of us get through our harder times.

After eighth grade, my two-year private school allotment ran out. My parents told me we couldn't afford the tuition any longer. I loved my teachers and the dance program, and had actually started to make a few friends at Fieldston by then. So I asked Mom and Dad if I could try getting a professional acting job in New York to pay for another year myself. It was a crazy idea—that I could make a lot of money quickly by acting—but my parents told me to go for it.

Mom took me to my first audition. Miraculously, I booked it, a commercial for the National Dairy Board. I was a featured ballerina in a group of dancers. But almost every identifiable part of me fell to the cutting room floor except for a brief glimpse of the bun on top of my head, a quick shot of my arm, and (debatably) my foot. I was crushed about being cut out but soon realized the job was a huge blessing regardless.

Over time, I made enough from residuals from that single thirty-second spot to cover another year of private education. But because the money didn't quite come in soon enough, I wound up enrolling for ninth grade in the public school in Rye, where we'd just moved. Nevertheless, the milk-ad money turned out to be just what I needed as a young actor. It paid for professional head shots and travel expenses for meetings for the next couple of years. At age fourteen I was signed by the William Morris Agency. My parents were thrilled.

Dad helped me learn lines. Mom weighed in on clothes (though we fought about short skirts) and sometimes drove me to Manhattan for auditions. Finally I started appearing in more commercials—for Stridex pads, Pizza Hut, and o.b. tampons (Mom didn't seem to mind that I was talking about my period in front of the whole world, and *that* was shocking). My senior year I was cast in an ABC Afterschool Special called *Stood Up*, based on a true story about a girl whose prom date was a no-show and she sued him. I played the bad girl, Vanessa, who got to go to the dance. In one scene I rode off on a motor scooter with the young man I'd stolen, glaring at the jilted girl, my hair flapping in the wind.

I applied to colleges in the beginning of my senior year—nine of them, because I worried most would reject me. I sat at Mom and Dad's typewriter (newly upgraded to electric!) and pounded out each application individually. My parents helped me craft my essays, and proofread every page. My mother came with me for on-campus interviews and shared my enthusiasm when the letter of acceptance arrived from Northwestern University outside of Chicago.

After I left home in 1989, tensions with Mom subsided. We needed space between us so we could miss each other. I told my agent in New York I wanted to focus on getting a college education, and my mother respected that. I'd be taking classes in the history of drama and doing behind-the-scenes crew work as well as acting. But I'd also be taking basic subjects like astronomy, German, and macroeconomics.

I was surprised that extracurricular activities at Northwestern were even more competitive than the showbiz scene in New York. I wasn't cast much when I was a freshman or during the first part of my sophomore year. Despite trying out for almost everything, I was mostly relegated to sewing costumes and focusing lights onstage. But the behind-the-scenes work gave me an appreciation for how much effort it takes to launch a production.

ONE AFTERNOON IN THE FALL of my sophomore year, I had no idea that I was on the verge of stepping onto a path that would alter the rest of my life.

My friend Abby, a fellow student in the middle of an internship in a casting office in Chicago, stopped me in the hall of the theater building. She told me that Steve Martin was starring in a remake of the old classic *Father of the Bride*. The producers were searching nationwide to fill the role played originally by seventeen-year-old Elizabeth Taylor. The planned lead in the new version, Phoebe Cates, had dropped out to have a baby.

I figured I had no chance of getting the part, so there was no need to stress about just another audition. Although I had a boyfriend, being a bride or even playing one was the furthest thing from my mind. I was nineteen and had just told my agent to back off for four years. *But what the hell,* I thought, *it might be a fun adventure for an afternoon.* I told Abby I would go to the meeting.

My head hurt that day. Maybe I was dehydrated. Maybe I was hungover. I almost didn't go. And then that mom-voice inside me whispered, *Maybe it'll be a great story one day!* Besides, I'd never taken the El from the campus in Evanston to Chicago before, and I wanted to see if I could figure out the train system.

I didn't get lost, I had fun reading the two scenes in the meeting, and I found my way back to campus. *Done.* I didn't even tell anyone else I'd gone.

But then, surprisingly, Abby phoned to say I had a callback, in LA. So I had to call my agent and parents and fill them in. Everyone was delighted. I skipped classes for a day, flew to California on the studio's dime, read with the director, Charles Shyer, and got invited to a separate meeting with Steve Martin. It went smoothly, despite my nerves about acting with one of my favorite comedians. As I left, Steve told me in front of Charles that I'd done well, especially under intimidating circumstances. I thought, *No matter what happens, someday I can tell my kids that once upon a time Steve Martin gave me a compliment.*

After I returned to campus, my agent, Jen, called from New York to tell me that I hadn't gotten the part—*Duh,* I thought—and she hadn't been told why.

I wondered if I even wanted to be an actor anymore. I was tired of other people calling the shots for me, telling me no. Maybe I needed a more reliable profession. I toyed with transferring into Northwestern's journalism school. My parents thought that was a terrific idea.

So did I, until Hollywood beckoned again. I learned later that the producers were having so much trouble casting the role, they went back and looked at old tapes of people they'd already dismissed. In bed with the flu, Charles's partner, Nancy Meyers, saw something in my audition she hadn't seen before. Now they wanted me to read once more with Steve Martin, as well as (gasp) Diane Keaton, in a full-on screen test.

Who needs a reliable profession?

I skipped class again and flew back to LA. Reading with me off camera, Steve was calm and kind, and Diane's quirky, self-deprecating smile put me at ease. When it was over, Nancy told me, "You'll be hearing from us sooner rather than later."

The next couple of days back in Chicago passed in slow motion. I could think of nothing else. Coincidentally, Mom, Jay, and Ash were visiting me at school for the weekend, and all we talked about was *what if.* We couldn't help ourselves. I imagined my dream becoming a reality. *A great role. A huge Hollywood movie. Incredible actors—people I've always looked up to.* And then I fought with myself. *It's just a dangling carrot. The chances are still really slim.*

Aren't they?

WE YEARNED FOR DISTRACTION AND went to Chicago to see a play with my boyfriend, Mike. I heard not a word of the first act. At intermission I called my agent again from a pay phone in the lobby.

"You got it!" Jen said.

"Shut up!" I yelled. I nodded to my mother, next to me. She screamed. We jumped up and down and collected an audience of our own. Mom hugged strangers.

I called my dad from the same phone and told him the news, and we skipped the second half of the play. All the way home, we sang the Blues Traveler's song "But Anyway" as loudly as we could out of the open-air windows of Mike's Jeep. It was a great stress release. We didn't talk. We were all in shock.

Back in my dorm room that night, I looked at all the recently unpacked crates of books, clothes, and pictures that were supposed to accompany me through my sophomore year. I'd hoped for a chance like this since I was a girl, but suddenly I was scared. I was grateful my mother was there with me to hold my hand and encourage me to take deep breaths.

The phone rang. It was Nancy Meyers. She congratulated me, told me that I needed to book myself a first-class ticket to Los Angeles for the next morning, and said she'd pay me back. (It was more than I'd ever put on my college credit card.) I hadn't realized I would have to leave so soon. She asked to speak to my mom.

"I just want you to know," she said, mother to mother, "there are a lot of crazy people in Hollywood, but Charles and I are not two of them. We don't do drugs. We're parents ourselves, and we'll treat Kim like a daughter. We'll take care of her."

I don't know if it had yet occurred to my mom that she was sending me into a potentially dangerous situation, but the call was reassuring to all of us. Nancy never suggested that Mom or Dad should fly out with me. She never spelled out exactly how long I'd be living in California. I was going alone. But not unprepared, as Mom assured me that night. All those years of auditions in New York City, my growing pains at Fieldston, and my recoveries from real and pro-verbial belly flops over time had strengthened me more than I realized. Mom knew that. At least she made me think she did.

SHOOTING THE MOVIE WAS THE hardest and most ex-hilarating work I'd ever done. The days were long, usually fifteen-plus hours at a time, with often less than a twelve-hour turnaround from leaving the sound stage or location to starting over the next day. I was by myself in an unfamil-iar city in a high-profile film. The pressure was exhausting. Everyone on the set was friendly and supportive, but the stress and lack of sleep made me sick several times.

My nightmares were so vivid I'd wake up sobbing and terrified. Some made sense. Others baffled me.

I was hanging off a cliff. Every branch I grabbed to save myself was too thin, and broke. . . . Steve Martin was hack-ing his own face with a razor blade. . . . I flapped my arms

*and flew away from my family, high over treetops. . . . I was
getting married. But I got ready before I was supposed to and
Mom was mad. . . . Mom got really sick. I was inconsolably
worried about her. . . .*

Finally my mother flew out to watch me work and to play
a small role in the filming of the wedding reception. It was
a comfort to see her, and the cast and crew were welcoming.
She loved her brief moments on camera, talking to Diane
in a crowd. She was there for the filming of my "first dance"
with the man I marry in the movie, George Newbern, who is
still a dear friend. When we finished one of the takes, I came
off the dance floor and found her crying.

"What's wrong?" I asked.

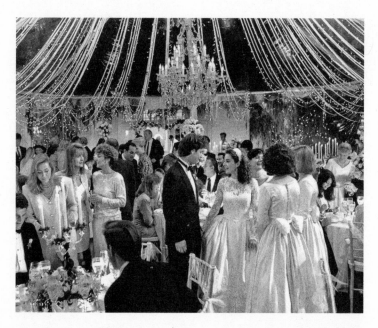

"I just hope you're this happy when you get married for real," she said.

Mom was often weepy then. She fretted over whether she'd been a good enough parent. She must have seen what I saw in my dreams—I was flying away from my family. We knew I would be forever changed by this experience, but we didn't yet know how. Maybe she worried it was too late to impart wisdom to me, or struggled to figure out what her role in my life was supposed to be now. We needed to become friends, but we weren't completely comfortable with that real-life role. We were both needy, so we alternated taking care of each other. She brought me warm soup and tea at the end of a long day. And I tried to reassure her.

"You're a great mom," I told her, again and again.

I took my family to Disneyland when my mother came back with my siblings to visit on a day off, and because Disney is the parent company to the movie studio, the Mouse not only paid for the tour of the park but gave us a private guide. We went to the head of every line, got free hot dogs, and felt like royalty. I bought a box of stationery and then accidentally left it in one of the cars on Space Mountain.

"Let's go back and get another one," Mom said, and she took off toward the other side of the park. Ash, Jay, and I followed her. When we got to the shop, a chain blocked the door and a sign told us they'd closed. We started to walk away. But then my mom stopped.

"Wait," she said. She turned back and climbed over the

chain. I marveled at her tenacity and followed her. We noticed a dim light inside the shop. I knocked on the door, and a woman saw me. As she walked our way, my mother whispered, "I'm gonna make up a story." I'd seen that look on her face before: impish, mischievous.

When the door opened, Mom wrung her hands and wove a charming tale. That is, she lied.

"Oh, hello! So sorry to bother you. We bought stationery here as a present for a friend and we lost it on Space Mountain and we're never going to be able to get it back because"—here came the hint of unspeakable sorrow—"we can't ever come back to Disneyland. *Ever*." With that, the store reopened just long enough to provide us with a new box. Though we offered to pay for it, the woman gave it to us for free.

"This really *is* the most magical place on earth," Mom told the woman, making her day. We giggled the whole way home, and I clutched my stationery, appreciating it all the more.

Father of the Bride *was* almost an instant classic. The Monday after the opening weekend, I got a call at home in New York from Jeffrey Katzenberg, who was then the head of Disney's motion picture division.

"Congratulations!" he cheered. "It's a hit!"

· · ·

I WENT FROM FEELING INVISIBLE at Northwestern to being the most recognizable person on campus. My picture was on the cover of *USA Today* and *People* magazine, and I was a guest on national programs like *The Tonight Show*. Wherever I went, people stopped me. Boys I'd never met showed up from other parts of the country at my dorm room. Women everywhere told me stories of their own weddings, and fathers reminisced about playing basketball with their daughters. I took pictures and signed autographs. Life was indeed very different.

MORE THAN A YEAR LATER, in July 1992, I invited my mom to accompany me on the press junket for the film's release in Japan. We flew first-class, all expenses paid, and felt completely spoiled by everything Japan Airlines offered: a hot towel, tube socks, a kimono, and chocolate fudge sundaes. We toasted with our orange juice in champagne glasses and made friends with the flight attendants.

We had connecting rooms in a lavish Tokyo hotel, and splurged on in-room massages. We called my dad direct on separate phones in our rooms and had him conference us in so we could all talk at the same time. In a sushi restaurant, Mom charmed a man at our table so much that he swiped a set of sake cups for her. We couldn't believe what we were being given (or being allowed to take), and no one celebrated it more than my mother. Her enthusiasm kept me going.

I had a lot of promotional work to do, and I was drained. On one particularly long and grueling day, I had to be a judge in the Best Father of the Bride Contest. But judgment was what I'd lacked in agreeing to be part of the show in the first place.

In the script, they would teleport me magically from California to Tokyo. When I appeared, I would recite the one phrase they'd taught me in Japanese. Roughly translated: "Where in the world am I?"

They put me in a short white Vera Wang dress, I guess to highlight that I was the movie bride. I was pushed onstage, without a translator, in front of a large audience including reporters.

The host seemed to welcome me at first. He rattled off a few sentences in Japanese and thrust the microphone in my face. That was my cue, so I said my line as best I could. The audience laughed. *Success.*

But then he kept jabbering and held the mic out to me again. I had no idea what to say. He added something else, maybe about how I was speechless. The audience roared. It was as if I were the subject of a comedy roast but didn't understand any of the jokes about me. Finally a producer in the wings beckoned. I waved and walked offstage with a big smile plastered on my face, but feeling embarrassed and confused.

I didn't have to say a word to my mom. As soon as I made it out of the spotlight, she responded with certainty about what to do. "Get her a bourbon!" she snapped at our guide, who hurried away to look for it backstage.

I was twenty years old and had only ever smelled bourbon. I didn't really want any. But in an instant, all the unwritten mother/daughter rules we'd previously established dissolved (rule one being never drink alcohol in front of Mom or Dad). Suddenly we were contemporaries. *So this is what she's like,* I thought, *when she's not trying to be a parent.*

We went out to a club together that night, danced and flirted with people, and laughed about how awful the day had been. My relationship with my mother began to shift. She was still Mom. But she was becoming my friend. I couldn't wait to get to know her better.

4

Before she met my father in 1964, Mom broke up with her previous boyfriend, in part because of the assassination of John F. Kennedy. She was a student in Paris at the time, homesick and devastated by the president's death. During a transatlantic phone call, her potential husband— a handsome, athletic business whiz, adored by her stockbroker father—didn't seem to empathize with her grief. It was one of the first signs that their relationship was rocky. They parted months later.

She met my dad at the perfect time, when she was ready to fall in love with someone quite different. She saw something in Gurney Williams that her father did not. When my dad formally asked George Payne for Mom's hand in marriage, my grandfather hardly knew what to say. Dad learned later that Grandpa was more than perplexed by the skinny liberal journalist sitting in front of him and was lamenting what might have been.

Like Mom after the Kennedy assassination, and like many Americans, I felt deep grief and isolation on September 11, 2001. I had been enjoying life. *Father of the Bride* had led to other film and television roles, most recently as a series regular on the ABC TV show *According to Jim*. But that day, as I sat immobile on my couch in Santa Monica, California, watching scenes of destruction and death, my work, my little house on the beach, and all the things in it didn't matter. Life, so very fragile, became simple. I prayed that my family and friends were all right.

My mother had gone back to work by then, as a fundraiser in New York City for Memorial Sloan Kettering Cancer Center. Our relationship was as strong as ever. Both of us were working hard and traveling a lot. We talked every couple of weeks or so, but I didn't know her daily schedule. Her office was about four miles from Ground Zero, and I wondered if maybe she'd had a meeting downtown. Friends of mine lived and worked all over Manhattan. Any of them could have been close to the attacks.

I worried about Ash, too. A budding actress, she spent a lot of time in the city, and she had been prepping that morning for an audition. And I thought about my brother, Jay, who at that time was training in California to become a firefighter. How many people with his brave commitment to rush toward danger had died that day?

Where was everyone?

There was no way to know. Phone lines were jammed. I felt helpless. By the time I walked away from my TV hours later, four hijacked jets had crashed and thousands had lost their lives.

I stepped outside onto my small front porch. The California sun sparkled on the Pacific beyond an empty beach at the end of my street. The city was unusually quiet. No planes rumbled overhead toward LAX. No traffic choppers whirred above the freeways. My neighbor appeared with his dog on a leash. We had occasionally traded hellos on the street. But on that day, without saying a word, we hugged.

Within hours, thankfully, I knew that everyone I loved was safe. But, driven by my vulnerability, I began to yearn to find someone to be by my side during future disasters, failures, or fears in the night. Someone who could celebrate success with me, laugh, listen, and understand me. I wonder now if Mom had been feeling the same way when she'd met my quirky and steadfast father.

I knew at the time that this was more of a wish than a plan, and I wasn't sure that it was realistic. Conversations with guys in LA, mostly actors, never delved much beneath the surface. I didn't fully trust them.

Enough. I wanted what my parents had: a stable, loving relationship. My wish became a prayer. A couple of weeks later, I wrote something like this on a scrap of notepaper:

I am ready to meet my life partner. I know this person is out there. Thank you, God, Universe, Higher Power, for protecting him and helping him to have a good day today. Help him to rest well tonight. Thank you for working out a way for us to find each other.

I rolled the paper into a tiny cigarette-sized cylinder and jammed it into a purple ceramic prayer jar with a cork lid by my bed. I never needed to reread it. At night, in the mornings, in the car driving to work, it became my mantra, a continuous song in my heart.

I am ready. Bring us together. Open his eyes. Help him find me.

And then, not five weeks after I began asking for divine matchmaking, a country singer named Brad Paisley woke up on his tour bus thinking of me. He swears this had never happened to him before.

He'd seen *Father of the Bride* nine years earlier with his girlfriend. When she broke up with him, he was devastated. Later she tried to reconcile. But Brad was conflicted. On the anniversary of their first date, he went to see *Father of the Bride, Part II* by himself. He hoped that if he and his ex were fated to be together, she'd have the identical idea and show up for the same show, ensuring that their lives were inexorably entwined. Brad is an idealist. A romantic.

Fortunately for me, she was neither. He went on to write a song about his great disappointment:

Hollywood never fails to make a sequel
For each and every movie that does well.
Why can't love be more like that,
Where the best ones get a second chance?
And that way though you're gone,
It wouldn't be that long
Till I'd see you in Part Two.

Through all of his pain, Brad didn't give a thought to Annie, the young bride on the screen. He pined after the girl who didn't show.

But years later, when he woke up after an overnight bus ride to Nashville from a Halloween concert in Kansas, he was suddenly determined to find me.

As he drove his truck past Opryland on the way back to his bachelor pad, he called the only person he knew well in Los Angeles. He hoped that Peter Tilden, a radio personality and writer, might be able to connect the two of us.

Brad was clueless about who I really was. Single? Married? No idea. But his plan had formed quickly. As his opening line, he was going to ask me if I'd appear in a music video for the song "Part Two." This was a little lie. He had no real plans to shoot it.

He was lucky. Peter knew my manager at the time, Tammi Chase. Brad reached her before he pulled into his driveway. Minutes later, the phone rang in my car as I was on my way home from a funeral.

"I just talked to the cutest guy," Tammi said. "A country singer. You're totally gonna date him."

"What?"

"He's got the coolest story to tell you. He said he wants you in a music video, but I think you guys are going to date. He's got a southern accent!"

Later that day, intrigued, I dialed Brad on his cell phone from my house. He picked up right away and began relaying *his* version of the *Father of the Bride* story. As he went through all the details, I tried to ask a question. He stopped me.

"No, I went to the seven-thirty show by myself, and when she didn't turn up, I bought a second ticket for the nine-thirty," he said. "Pay attention!" I loved his sassy humor and the way he made fun of me right away. We talked for a long time. He tossed off a few words about the video he wanted to make, but quickly the conversation turned to other things—life in Tennessee versus California, our families, and relationships. We were both children of long-standing marriages and hoped to follow our parents' examples. We exchanged email addresses, traded messages, and talked again a few days later. I was dying to meet this guy in person. Was he the answer to my prayer? We stayed in touch during the next couple of weeks, each conversation more interesting than the last.

We had a lot to learn from our differences, especially our tastes in music. I'd never listened to country. My family listened to the Beatles, Top Forty, classical music, Broadway soundtracks, and even the Yale singing group the Whiffen-poofs from my dad's time in college. I hadn't heard of the Opry, and thought Brad said he was going to perform "at the opera" *(was it his accent?)* when he first told me about the original home of country music.

A few weeks later, Brad came to LA for work and I asked him to dinner. At the restaurant in Marina del Rey, he excused himself to the bathroom while I was in the middle of telling a story. He was reserved and a little nervous in person. We had a pleasant couple of dates, but I didn't sense the humor that had been there over the phone. I wondered if we had the connection I'd thought we did. I told him I wanted to proceed cautiously.

"That's totally fine," he said. "I get it. I like you. I like spending time with you. I don't know what this relationship is supposed to be, but I think we're meant to be in each other's lives. Maybe just as friends." He was calm, confident, understanding. "If you want to go to dinner again some-time," he told me, "I'll fly to wherever you are to make it happen." There was no game playing here. No drama. It was really attractive.

So I TOOK HIM AT his word. I didn't make a commitment to him, and we stayed in touch. In late December I decided to accept his dinner invitation. I was going to be in New

York and thought it might be fun to meet him in my home state.

"How's December twenty-eighth?" I asked, not knowing that was the same date Brad had first gone out with his old girlfriend exactly ten years earlier.

Bad weather on the day of our date meant that Brad's flight was rerouted to White Plains, just fifteen minutes from my parents' home. So I invited them to join us.

I thought the dinner at an Italian restaurant went well. There was one awkward moment when Brad seemed to forget my dad was talking and leaned in to whisper something in my ear. But overall, the conversation flowed. Mom giggled easily, though she was mostly quiet while my father and Brad got more serious, talking about music and religion. In what almost seemed like a Freudian slip of a move, when we left the restaurant Dad accidentally pulled away from the curb before Brad could get into the car. We all laughed it off, but the truth was, my father was a little nervous. Maybe he sensed there was a lot at stake.

"Wow," he said to my mom later, when my parents were alone, meaning he was impressed.

"Yeah, can you believe that?" Mom said, meaning she was sure it wouldn't last.

Ironically, although my mother didn't notice it, Brad was in some ways like her last boyfriend before Dad. Brad had a business degree and a solid career plan. He was talented, successful, self-assured. He knew how to ride a horse, drive a truck, and shoot a gun. He was a guy's guy. My mother's father would have been thrilled.

Maybe Brad was too quick to assume he didn't have to work hard to impress her. He was casual in front of her, and maybe she was expecting more formality. In West Virginia, Brad grew up drinking filtered water. When I offered him a glass straight out of the tap in our kitchen in New York ("the cleanest water in the country," Mom always insisted), he joked, "Why don't you just pee in it?"

Maybe this boyish humor distracted my mother from his talent and charm. Or perhaps she just wasn't ready to face the reality that her first child might start her own family all too soon. She assumed I'd move on, perhaps the way she had many years earlier.

She may also have sensed the truth, which was that I was still unsure. *Was there enough there between the two of us for me to really commit to a long-distance relationship? I know I said I was ready to meet the one, God, but is this him?* I called Brad once we'd both returned to our homes after a couple of days together in New York. I let him know that I was still reticent. His reaction surprised me. He got fired up, and for the first time I saw his passion.

"I don't want to take *anything* away from your life," he said, his voice louder than I'd ever heard it. "I only want to *add* to your life." He told me he'd wait until I decided how I wanted to move forward.

And then he went off and wrote "Little Moments." We

now joke that this is the song that got him married. He called and played it for me over the phone:

I'll never forget the first time that I heard
That pretty mouth say that dirty word...

It was the *F*-word. I knew right away that he was referring to the first time I said it in front of him, right after he told me he didn't curse. I wanted to see what he would do, if the southern gentleman could handle a northern woman's potty mouth. At the time, he chuckled in surprise. But he was fine.

The lyrics in "Little Moments" made me recognize Brad's insight about me for the first time. He'd written poetry from mere snapshots of our relationship, pictures I never would've remembered because they seemed insignificant at the time. Not only did he understand me, he appeared to accept and adore me as I was.

I invited him back to California. Over two days, everything changed. After that weekend and a few trips out on the road on the tour bus (ten guys and me!), I'd fallen in love with him.

As we walked on the pier in Marina del Rey one night, I pressed Brad about why he'd called me in the first place.

"I don't know," he said. "I just woke up with the clearest feeling that we were supposed to be in each other's lives." It seemed to both of us like divine intervention.

I called home and told Mom and Dad I'd never felt this way about someone before. They sounded startled. I could

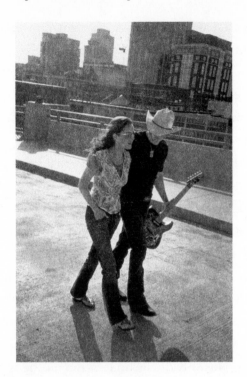

hear it in their voices. *Really? So soon?* My mother stifled her hesitation, apparently still thinking that my infatuation would fade. On the contrary, Brad and I started seeing each other whenever possible.

Eight months after we met, Tammi asked me to meet a photographer who was working on the pier Brad and I had walked on not long before.

I passed a few families and men at the railings, their fishing lines vanishing in the gray early evening light. *This is our pier,* I thought. I saw none of the tripods, reflectors, or bustle of a photo shoot. It felt strange to be there without Brad, who was in Tennessee (or so I thought).

And then suddenly, out from behind the public restrooms, he appeared. His hands were in his pockets. He looked like a casual angel. Then he pulled one hand out, and in it was a ring. No one around us knew what was happening. The fishermen ignored us. An older couple chased after their children.

Brad knelt on one knee and said, "So . . . will ya?"

"Will I *what*?"

"Will you marry me?"

"Yes!" I said, just as we heard someone flush a toilet.

"There go our lives," Brad said.

I giggled and knelt down on the dried-fish-gut-coated wooden slats with my fiancé, and we hugged. It was one of the happiest moments of my life.

Until I called home a few minutes later.

It began like a scene from *Father of the Bride*.

"I'm engaged! I'm getting married!" was something like what I shouted on the phone. Mom's stunned silence and then halting congratulations spoke volumes. She asked me if I was sure, and suggested that we didn't know each other well enough. Dad, sensitive to my mother's feelings, muted his enthusiasm. In fact, Brad had already discussed the upcoming proposal with him over the phone, unbeknownst to my mother and me. My father had told him that the decision was mine to make but that he would be supportive of both of us.

My conversation with my parents ended abruptly, and I knew Mom had left much unsaid. I was hurt and disappointed, and my excitement lost a little steam, but I down-played it. For one of the first times in my life, I was certain about what I was going to do in spite of my mother's disapproval. I felt as if there was no way I could *not* marry Brad.

The first time I saw my mother after I got engaged, she invited me to breakfast with my father but without Brad. We huddled in a booth at Joni's Coffee Roasters in Marina del Rey with several cups of coffee and eggs we hardly touched. As Dad sat silently next to her, Mom told me she was concerned. Brad and I didn't have enough in common. She couldn't understand why I thought he was the one. And on and on. It was a cross-examination and I was the defendant.

I fought hard for our choice, knowing that I couldn't show any weakness or hesitation. *I trust him. I love him. I need him. I want him to be my husband, Your Honor.*

"I know he may not be who you'd pick, Mom," I said.

She was crying by the time she and my dad dropped me off at my house in Santa Monica. Brad appeared on the porch to say hello, unaware of our breakfast conversation. I think my mother must have asked my father to take her away. She was probably embarrassed and didn't want to hurt Brad's feelings. Dad accelerated as she rolled her window down and waved manically with a big plastic smile on her face.

"What the heck was that?" Brad asked.

I shook my head. "I'm really sorry," I told him. There was no doubt he was wounded. But there was nothing he or I could do. At least for now, Mom had distanced herself from us. My choice was clear: my fiancé over her.

TWO AND A HALF MONTHS before the wedding, we got the news that Brad's aunt Rita had suffered a recurrence of breast cancer. She was to begin treatment soon after Christmas. Brad has a small family, and we needed to go home to support them. My parents had flown from New York to be in California for the holiday, now that all their kids lived there. But as Brad's betrothed, I knew the right thing for me to do was return with him.

We told Mom and Dad the news. Our plan was to stay with my family through early Christmas morning, then fly to West Virginia. To me, that was a fair compromise. But to my mother, whose anxiety had only grown, it was as though I'd said we were moving to Alaska and would never return. It was the first time any of Mom's three kids would break away from our tight-knit tribe to support someone else's family. It gutted her.

The following day, Brad and I drove to my parents' hotel. Mom sobbed on a lounge chair on the deck outside their room with my father next to her, comforting her. She had covered her face with a washcloth. She swiped it aside and looked at Brad. He held out his arms to hug her. She shrugged him off and stood up.

"No," she said, and went inside. I was mortified.

She continued to cry off and on for two days until we

left. This was not the "Go for it!" mother of my childhood. Her fear seemed out of proportion with our family "crisis." Adding to my pain, my father appeared to abandon me to take her side. Jay and Ashley tried to remain neutral and be sympathetic listeners.

The break with my parents had some silver linings. It fortified my bond with Brad. And at the height of the flood tide of tears, he and my father connected in a brief phone conversation, commiserating about the women they loved as if they'd known each other for a long time.

"How's Kim doing?" my father asked.

"She's cryin'."

"Oh, man."

"How's Linda?" Brad asked.

"Crying."

WE ROSE EARLY ON CHRISTMAS morning, flew to West Virginia, and celebrated with Rita and the rest of the family. We were so glad we did. It was the last holiday when everyone in Brad's family would be together. His aunt died eleven months later.

That Christmas, a question began to nag at me, and it would persist even during some of the good times to come: *Is this extreme behavior somehow beyond her control? What in the world is going on with Mom?*

CHAPTER

5

After our wedding, Mom warmed to Brad. Maybe for the first time, she saw him through other people's eyes. Our friends and extended family had surrounded us in the Pepperdine chapel and sung, cheered, and spoken on our behalf. Maybe she realized that we were committed—there was no going back. Maybe it was the magic of the ceremony that healed the scars of the previous year, exorcised my mother's bitterness, and awakened more than just acceptance of her son-in-law. She loved him.

Brad and I were happy to forget the discord during our engagement and celebrate the harmony of our marriage. I went back to work on the sitcom; Brad toured and finished a new album. He wrote the song "That's Love," with the lyric "You'll say 'I like it when your mother comes to visit us.' That's not a lie, that's love." It made my mom laugh.

We imagined that the tough times with her were behind us.

But the challenges of her new job at the Michael J. Fox Foundation were just beginning. Recently she'd been having trouble reading as quickly as she used to, and sometimes she struggled to find the right word when she spoke. It wasn't a persistent enough problem that she shared it with anyone, but it did affect her confidence on the first day of work. She hid her fear as best she could and shook hands with her new colleagues, offered hugs, and laughed to cover her nerves.

In many ways, she was at the top of her abilities. She'd already proven herself to be a brilliant fundraiser at Sloan Kettering. Headhunters had sought her. She'd happily left the world-class cancer center to become director of development at the far smaller Fox Foundation, to help champion an effort to cure Parkinson's disease. Its staff was smart and idealistic, on a bold mission to fight a neurological illness that affects a million people in this country alone, including Fox himself.

She was about to turn their idea of fundraising upside down. It wasn't just about collecting dollars, she would tell them. It was about offering rare opportunities to people they would come to know and often genuinely adore. She realized that she was by far the oldest person in the office and soon emerged as a mentor. "It's never an insult to ask someone for too much money," she told her protégés. "We are giving them a gift, an opportunity to participate in this amazing organization." She knew philanthropists were more than eager to be generous.

I admired her technique: Get to know a prospect well after many conversations and, best of all, visits. Love them. Love what they love. Mom was the master of the hardest part of the job, The Ask (i.e., "We'd like you to consider pledging a million dollars"). She taught everyone how to do it.

She walked into each donor visit with excitement and high expectations. She sparkled, warmed up the conversation, and spoke from her heart. Then came The Ask. The next step was key. She let the request hang in the air, maintaining eye contact and waiting without saying a word for as long as it took to get a response. Inexperienced fundraisers often filled the silence too soon, apologizing or scrambling to lower the amount. Not Mom.

When donors agreed to a gift, my mother knew how to show gratitude and appreciate one of the best moments a good life has to offer: giving to a good cause. Back in the office, she celebrated the win with everyone on the team.

Mom followed up every meeting with a personal and heartfelt thank-you note. She insisted on paying attention to small details. Her finishing touch was a gold paper clip— the final version of every important letter or proposal was always secured with one, like a gilded ribbon on a present.

She was also a friend to her co-workers. One day she went looking for a member of her team and found her in the cramped supply closet, one of the only private spaces in the small office. The woman was organizing everything, and she was crying. Mom closed the door enough so that they were alone, and hugged her. With no room to sit down, they stood together, surrounded on two sides by shelves full of gala invitations, envelopes, and toner cartridges. Mom listened and empathized as her colleague privately shared a non-work-related problem. The two of them reorganized everything, alphabetizing and moving boxes from one shelf to another and back, until her friend was ready to put on a professional stiff-upper-lip face and return to office work. The care my mother offered ran deep and was one of her strongest traits.

But the new job highlighted increasing challenges. In one meeting, her boss, co-founder Debi Brooks, laid into the development team about their lack of attention to forecasting and budget. It was fair criticism aimed squarely at my mother.

Another problem was that on expeditions with Debi in the constant quest for new funding, Mom got nervous behind the wheel of their rental car, afraid she would get lost or cause an accident. So she delegated *up*, asking her superior to do the driving.

She told no one but Dad about her growing dread that she couldn't handle important parts of her job. She was having trouble sleeping again, and fretted about the workday to come. Dad woke up one winter night and knew without opening his eyes that Mom wasn't in bed with him. He found her in the guest room with the door open.

"I don't know how to run a meeting," she told him. In some ways, this wasn't a surprise. Dad had seen her suffer with simpler tasks, such as learning some of the basic facts about Parkinson's. He worried that she'd taken on too much. My parents sat together on their old saggy bed, the first one they'd slept on as a newly married couple. Dad scratched her back to soothe her, and suggested starting with the basics.

"Thank them," he said. "Talk about what the meeting is for. You'll get better at this the more you do it."

ONE AFTERNOON IN 2004, MY father was sitting on the living room couch when my mother came down the stairs naked. She was puzzled.

"Where's my—" she said, and stopped. Mom wasn't the kind of person to walk around the house without clothes, even if just the two of them were at home. They stared at each other for a second, then started laughing. Dad got up, hugged her, and led her back upstairs to get a robe. He was less concerned than amused.

During one of her fundraising trips to LA, Mom and I met for a drink at Shutters in Santa Monica, close to my house. A damp ocean breeze rolled over the deck, where we sat looking out to the dark beach just yards away. Far from the office, Mom was able to relax and have fun. And I was relieved that the two of us seemed to be getting closer again.

We ate Cape Cod potato chips at a small table next to a few other patrons. I ordered a vodka and cranberry juice. Mom probably sipped an apple martini. She'd given up bourbon on the rocks in favor of the sweeter green cocktail, and joked that it looked healthier.

"Loaded with vitamin C," she said, and winked.

She asked me about work, and I filled her in on the farm Brad and I had just bought in Tennessee.

"Deer, wild turkeys, and some Canada geese live on the land. There's a soulful old house and a pond and a tiny graveyard from the late eighteen hundreds. Apparently an albino buck roams the woods nearby, though we've never seen it," I rambled on.

Finally Mom brought up what was really on her mind.

"Something kind of weird has been happening with me lately," she said. One day back home, when she pulled out her checkbook to pay for groceries at Stop & Shop, she forgot how to write the numbers. Another time, while people waited behind her in a line, she struggled to sign her name.

Odd, I thought. But almost immediately I dismissed it.

"That kind of thing happens to everyone from time to time," I said. "You need more sleep." I wasn't going to let her concerns get blown out of proportion again, and I didn't want to tell her that I was worried the new job was too demanding.

To our right, we could see the Santa Monica Pier, and part of the Ferris wheel Jay and I used to ride, its lights blinking as it turned.

"You need to relax more," I added. "You're putting too much stress on yourself."

She nodded. "You're probably right."

BUT BACK IN RYE, NEW YORK, at an annual exam with my mother's internist in July 2004, there was just this one thing. Mom at sixty-one appeared to be healthy in most respects. Her weight was 130, her blood pressure normal at 120/70. She registered fine cholesterol numbers, and previous issues with migraines and asthma had been resolved. Even her neurological exam was not unusual. But Silvio Ceccarelli, M.D., noted in her record that she had struggled a little with a few brief mental exercises he'd given her in his office. Dad was there to watch.

"Count backward from a hundred by sevens," the doctor said. "Like this: a hundred, ninety-three, eighty-six, and so on, okay?"

"Oh! All right!" Mom slapped her thighs as though firing a starting gun. "Let's see . . . eighty-six. So, by sevens . . . eighty-six, seventy . . . nine!" She aced a few more numbers, but then asked to hear the question again, and wasn't able to produce more than one or two correctly after that. There was a false calm in the office. Mom looked to my father and shrugged, forcing a smile.

The next task: "Who is the current vice president?"

"Yes," she said with a grimace. She knew that one. They followed politics closely. The vice president was a Republican. She hadn't voted for him. She could picture his face. She patted her chest. "The name. The name . . ." Silence.

"Dick?" the doctor prompted after a few seconds.

"Cheeney!" she said. "Choney. You know. Cheney!"

"Yay!" Dad said.

Dr. C. scribbled more notes and referred her—"if you want to pursue this"—to a neurologist in the same practice, for further examination. That specialist ruled out Lyme disease but wasn't sure what else might be wrong. Maybe nothing.

For several months after that visit, Mom and Dad sought to get long-term-care insurance. But the paperwork filled out by both physicians expressed a slight concern about the well-being of her brain. Nerves crippled her as she fumbled through intelligence drills given to her by an insurance company over the phone. There would be no safety net of coverage.

For months, Mom and Dad stopped further tests and avoided talking about their concerns with us. After all, Mom was still able to work, and held hope that the stress she felt would subside and her mind would clear. She didn't want to alarm the family. I think she was fearful that if she continued to seek other opinions, someone would discover that she wasn't as smart as we all thought she was, or that it was her own fault she couldn't get her stress under control. My parents never talked with each other about the possibility of dementia.

But her difficulties on the job were rising to a level impossible to ignore. She had to acknowledge to her colleagues that it took longer to write proposals to donors. That she wasn't as comfortable as other foundation directors when speaking to large groups. That it was hard to keep up with the administrative parts of the work in the office. One supervisor's evaluation reported that Mom found it challenging to get her voice heard among her peers, and that often she gave up trying to be heard at all.

In the fall of 2004, she asked to be reassigned to lesser duties, at lower pay. "She faced the uncertainty of change with grace," her supervisor wrote. Just a few months later, she and Dad decided they could no longer bear the uncertainty. They set out on a new and more serious quest for a diagnosis.

It began with PET and CT scans. Those revealed mild cerebral atrophy—some of her brain cells were withering away. The scans looked almost normal, her latest neurologist, Nancy Nealon in New York City, told Dad. That meant that, like others before her, the doctor couldn't explain the loss. Dr. Nealon set up the most intensive mental testing my mother had ever had, stretching out over three months, from August until October 2005. The extent of this further analysis was kept secret from me at Mom's request until later that year.

I DIDN'T KNOW THE WEIGHT of the burden they were carrying when my parents showed up in Tennessee for

Christmas with beautifully wrapped presents to put under the tree. Given our recent history, I'd worried about their visit. But my anxiety revolved around wanting Mom's approval of my new home and my new life with Brad. I wanted her to love the way we were living, to feel comfortable in our home, to admire our Christmas tree. I wrestled with getting a real one or a fake.

My mother had always placed a lot of emphasis on the tree. It was the centerpiece for every Christmas. She adored living, aromatic evergreens and thought synthetic versions were tacky. But artificial ones were more practical. They could be reused every year, and the needles didn't scatter all over the floor.

In a stab at further independence, I opted for fake. I fussed over every decoration and detail. I made sure the smell of warm apple cider greeted them when they knocked on the door.

Mom was dressed in her typical Christmas "costume," which had evolved over the years to include more and more elements: the pilly, oversized red sweater, woven from thick cotton yarn with a big Santa face on the front. Dark blue socks splattered with red and green wreaths. Seasonal earrings, big red ornaments that dangled beneath her lobes. A golden sleigh bell tied around her neck with a red silk string.

Mom cheered as she walked through the door, and handed me a pair of my own red-and-white striped "elf" socks with white fur sewn around the top. She pulled out gifts wrapped in gold paper, finished with green ribbons curled at the ends. I handed her a mug of cider.

Shortly after they settled in, Dad whispered to me that he and Mom needed to "talk to the kids." *Oh, God,* I thought. *They hate the tree. They hate everything about Christmas at my home.*

"Brad too?" I asked. I flashed back again to our dramatic California Christmas.

"Yes, he's welcome," Dad said. *(Phew.)* Jay was working in California and wasn't scheduled to fly in until the next day. Apparently Dad's urgency overrode the fact that not all of their children were there.

Is it my in-laws? While my parents and Brad's seemed to get along just fine, I worried that maybe Mom and Dad were having some problem with them. Though Brad's parents, Sandy and Doug, were also somewhere in the house, as well as Neal, Ashley's future husband, my father didn't invite any of them to come upstairs to our bedroom. I was concerned our covert meeting would hurt their feelings, but I didn't say anything.

Ash and I sat on the red comforter on Brad's and my queen-sized bed. My mother was on the floor next to my dad. Brad stood.

Mom's mood had deflated, and she stared at the carpet like a child who'd just gotten into trouble. Dad took a breath.

"We've been trying for a while now to figure out what's been going on with your mom," he said calmly. "In October we got a preliminary diagnosis."

I thought it was just anxiety, sleep deprivation. They got a diagnosis? Two months ago? I sensed Dad had been rehearsing this speech.

My mother glanced at us. *You're not gonna like this,* her expression seemed to say. She shook her head and focused back on the floor. My father held her hand.

"Primary progressive aphasia, or PPA," he said. "*Primary* means that a communication problem—aphasia—is the first sign of the disease. *Progressive* means it's going to get worse. Many stroke victims experience aphasia, but often it's treatable. From what we heard, PPA isn't."

This has got to be a mistake, I thought. *Explainable. Fixable.* Mom looked up at Ash and me again and shook her head more slowly this time, as if she were reading our thoughts. *No,* she seemed to be saying. *It's not.*

"We can't begin to know how your mom's illness will progress. It varies a lot from patient to patient. But doctors predict that it'll be five to seven years before your mother will need a whole lot of help."

He was treading carefully, as though he knew Mom might detonate at any moment with sadness, anger, fear. In her emotional state, it was hard for her to do any of the talking. His speech was measured, unemotional, calm. I tried to absorb all of it, but denial and anger were taking over. *They're wrong. This doesn't make sense.*

"I want you to know that your mom and I are together in this, and we are closer than ever." He put his arm around my mother and pulled her to him. He seemed to be saying this more for her benefit than anyone else's. Ashley's face was crumpling. Mom choked back a sob, and tears rolled down her face. My sister moved from the bed to Mom's side. I flashed back to the last few months. They must have been agonizing secretly. I wondered why they hadn't told us, though it seemed irrelevant in the moment to ask the question out loud. But Dad went on to explain it.

He said, "Your mother hasn't been ready to share this information. She asked me to keep it private until she was ready. So that's why we're just telling you now. It's really important to her that you guard her privacy and not talk about this with people outside the family. She doesn't want sympathy. She doesn't want you to treat her any differently. She wants you to laugh with her about this as much as possible. And anything you need to say to one of us, you can say to both of us."

I stayed seated on the bed, not wanting to move. I felt that if I gave in to their sorrow I would be accepting that this was real, and I wasn't willing to do that yet. Finally I asked if we could invite Sandy, Doug, and Neal upstairs, and my mother agreed, somewhat reluctantly. We all crowded back into the room, more comfortable in that smaller private space than downstairs in the living room. Dad repeated the diagnosis and the request for discretion.

In a whole new way, we joined forces as one extended family on our farm. It was the first time my mother had allowed Brad's parents to see her vulnerable, and their kindness and support were healing.

"Well, I'll help you if you help me," Sandy said. "I can't keep track of anything these days. Maybe I have dementia, too!" We laughed, grateful for a release. Doug said they'd help my parents in any way they could, and he meant it.

AFTER CHRISTMAS, JAY, ASHLEY, AND I had different ways of dealing with the news. For the most part I stayed true to my mother's request for the time being, discussing her illness only with Brad and my siblings. I hoped it wasn't as bad as doctors were saying, and I figured we could deal with it when we needed to. I was much more comfortable distracting myself with work, our new puppy, Holler, and married life.

Because Jay was now a paramedic firefighter, he looked into Mom's medical data, trying to boil down her disease into numbers he could understand and use to help her. He also agreed not to talk about it outside the family.

Ashley dove into research in a way that no one else had the guts to. She wanted to live out the journey we were facing before it happened so that she could be better prepared when it came. Of the three of us, I found out later, she was alone in knowing about the extent of the testing while it was happening. My mother had asked her not to tell the rest of us. So she didn't.

Before Mom's first diagnosis, my sister read an article in the *New York Times* about people learning to recover their memories. She wrote to a specialist mentioned in the article, Dr. Gary Small at UCLA, and told him our mom's story, asking if she could see him. Amazingly, the doctor wrote back, agreeing to an appointment. But when Ash called my parents to tell them about it, they were furious. Had she forgotten? She wasn't supposed to be discussing my mother's health with anyone. They would not be going to the appointment. Ash called me, upset, and told me she'd "gotten in trouble" with Mom and Dad. I was frustrated and surprised that their reaction had been so strong against seeing another professional. It wasn't as if she'd told anyone who knew us personally. Mom was missing a potential opportunity to get more help.

But their reaction didn't prevent my sister from reading books on Alzheimer's (there weren't any on PPA). She joined a Yahoo! PPA support group and read through dozens of member questions, such as "What do I do when my wife tries to bite me?" She found an end-of-life specialist who helped paint a picture of dementia for her and told her that we needed to find out from my mother very specifically what she wanted in terms of care once she could no longer tend to herself.

"This is going to be brutal," the woman told my sister. "And your mom needs to think now about things like what she wants her care to be like once she can no longer swallow. Get her exact wishes in writing."

Ash was able to convince Mom and Dad to have a phone conversation with the specialist. But they were irritated with what the woman said and how she said it. She didn't elaborate and didn't ask many questions. The talk felt like a sermon from someone who thought she knew everything, and my parents didn't want to hear it. They didn't want to discuss end-of-life decisions. They had a different focus: taking the advice that Dr. Nealon had given them just before they left her office on the day of the diagnosis. "Enjoy each other while you can," she'd said. It wasn't enough, Ashley knew, but again she had to back off.

It's possible that despite these rejections, Mom learned to see my sister as her closest ally. Ashley alone—not my father—knew something about my mother's wishes about her care down the road. One day during the testing, my sister met Mom for lunch at La Bonne Soupe, an unpretentious New York bistro that served foods my mother loved: freshly baked bread and homemade soups. They finished the meal. Ash asked how it was going, and reluctantly my mother told her: not well. They sobbed.

Then Mom reached across the table and gripped my sister's hands.

"I don't ever want Daddy to take care of me," my mother cried. "Please. Please don't let that happen."

"I won't," Ash said.

WHAT MY FATHER HADN'T REVEALED to any of us at the farm over Christmas was that after they'd gotten the bad news in New York, they'd driven home to Rye that sunny day without saying a word, and they'd remained almost speechless as they went upstairs to their bedroom and lay down.

"Scout," he said eventually, "we'll get all the help we need so you can stay in this house. You won't ever have to leave home."

We were all making promises we would never be able to keep.

6

That spring, I discovered I was pregnant. And one of my first thoughts was *Oh, crap, how's Mom gonna react to this one?*

Brad and I sat alone at the back of his tour bus in the parking lot of a fair somewhere in the middle of the country. He had about three hours until showtime. We stared for two of those hours at the stick from a cheap pregnancy test. It had been hard enough to buy it secretly in a grocery store ten minutes away. Now two little pink lines confronted us, one faint, the other bright. They had to be a mistake. But the more we reread the instructions, Googled images of positive test results, and gawked at the accusatory stripes, the more the news sank in. This was happening—unplanned, unexpected. I guess it runs in the family.

How could it be? I'd been in Atlanta shooting the film *We Are Marshall*, and we hadn't even seen each—

Oh, wait. There was that one weekend I made that quick trip home. Whoops.

We stared at each other, disbelieving. We pledged to get more tests in the morning to confirm. There was some measure of excitement, since we knew we wanted to have kids one day. But we also felt overwhelmed, realizing that our lives had just veered in a whole new direction.

I couldn't suppress the feeling, no matter how ridiculous, that I was going to get in trouble with my parents. Mom would reject Brad again, or get upset with me for interrupting my career. *She might tell me I've ruined my life,* I thought. I braced myself for what I imagined might be a showdown.

It would unfold eight weeks into the pregnancy at Ashley's apartment on the West Side of Manhattan, where she was acting in a play. Waiting for Mom and Dad to arrive, Ash and I poured milk into champagne glasses and practiced how I would break the news. My newly enlarged pregnancy boobs hurt. I felt nauseated and fatigued. So when my parents arrived, I let Brad do all the talking, via Skype, from somewhere else on the road.

They sat, squinting at the laptop screen, straining to hear. It took a few seconds for them to understand.

"We're gonna have a baby," Brad repeated.

They pushed back from the screen and both stood up, looking to me. Dad's mouth opened wide; Mom covered her face with her hands. Their eyes were wet with tears and laughter. They were ecstatic.

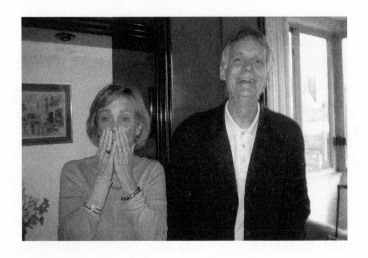

Relief!

New life was what we all needed to shift our focus from the other new life—the one we didn't want to imagine or embrace—that we were facing with Mom.

WE WERE STILL DENYING THE grim projections about her disease months later when we met in Chicago to get a second opinion.

My belly was just starting to protrude that October. Morning sickness had passed. The overwhelming smell of cocoa from the Blommer chocolate factory swirled around us as Jay, Ash, and I walked with our mother and father together to a specialist's office. It was a good omen. When we were kids, my father had made up stories during long road trips or at bedtime. We starred in all his tales, and whatever else they were about–kangaroos, bandits, motorcycles– each ended the same way: "... and they had freshly baked chocolate chip cookies and hot chocolate, and that was the end." Chocolate in any form was comforting evidence that everything turned out all right. Now we hoped that Dr. M.-Marsel Mesulam, the world's expert on primary progressive aphasia, would make it so.

A year had passed since Mom's first diagnosis. Ashley had stumbled on Dr. Mesulam's name when she read that he was the first to recognize PPA as a dementia separate from Alzheimer's disease (AD). He was director of the Cognitive Neurology and Alzheimer's Disease Center at Northwestern's Feinberg School of Medicine. We felt lucky to have gotten an appointment with him, and grateful that at least the family could be together for a rare reunion.

Few people outside the five of us knew that Mom was in trouble. At home, Dad helped hide her symptoms. He often edited her reports and letters for her job at the Fox Foundation. When she needed help in social settings, she signaled him with a worried glance or a touch on his arm. All of us had learned to patch up awkward silences with small talk during conversations. We knew it was unrealistic to believe that no one outside the inner circle noticed how Mom hesitated when she talked or made mistakes when she wrote. We hoped that the charade might end with this visit.

But our expectations were higher than that. Maybe her New York doctors had been wrong. Or if they were right, perhaps doctors here would tell us about a breakthrough—a pill, or maybe the news that researchers were on the verge of a major discovery.

We were giddy when we arrived at our hotel on the evening before the appointment. Because we talked about everything except why we were there, it felt like a vacation. We ordered pizza and beer, lounged on the double beds in our parents' room, and watched *Little Miss Sunshine*. I lay on my back and let Jay and Dad serenade my growing baby in two-part harmony. My mother—grandma-in-waiting—seemed surprisingly at ease.

But the next morning, our brief holiday was over. In the elevator to the doctor's office, Ash and I forced a joke or two. Mom was silent. My father and brother were stoic. A few older couples sat in the small waiting room. They looked bored. Had they been there many times before? Were they there for the same reason? *Are you giving us a glimpse of our future?* We studied them. *Are we going to be friends?* We never saw them again.

Dr. Mesulam invited Mom into his windowless office, where she and Dad sat down and the rest of us crowded in around them. He had a neatly trimmed grayish beard and was wearing a suit and tie, making him look professorial and somber. We had a lot of questions, but he wasn't ready to answer them.

"I'd like to evaluate Linda alone before we talk further," he said. In other words, the rest of us were not invited.

"See you in a minute," we said, or something generic like that. She looked small and scared as she sat there, trying to smile for us. We waved and gave her a thumbs-up. I hated to leave her alone.

But back in the waiting room, we exhaled and got real with each other. We'd been stifling our feelings around Mom. For the first time together away from her, we began checking each other for an emotional pulse. We focused on our father. None of us had been able to talk with him alone, in person or on the phone, in what felt like months.

"How are you?" I asked.

Dad knew we were well beyond small talk. He spoke rapidly in a whisper.

"I'm tired," he said. "Your mom is really challenged at work. We fight a lot more at home. She wants to do everything herself, but she just can't anymore. I want her to stop driving, but she's stubborn, and I don't know how to get the keys away from her."

We agreed that we needed to check in more often, but it was almost impossible. Increasingly, Mom insisted on being in on every phone call from Dad. Talking with us behind her back felt to my father like a betrayal, undermining the trust between them.

There was no time to challenge him. What seemed like seconds later, we were called back to Dr. Mesulam's office.

Someone had supplied enough chairs for all of us this time. Mom looked despondent. Dad didn't dare hold her hand, aware that she was trying not to cry for fear she'd look weak.

"I have confirmed the diagnosis," Dr. Mesulam said.

He went on to tell us everything we didn't want to hear.

Like the doctors in New York—he had studied their reports—he'd based his conclusion on the fact that Mom's difficulties had really begun with speaking and writing, hallmarks of aphasia. PPA first attacked the part of her brain behind her forehead. This frontotemporal area is primarily responsible for language. Her memory was healthy. That alone set her apart from people with AD, whose earliest symptom is usually forgetfulness.

Most people diagnosed with AD are over sixty-five. The first symptoms of frontotemporal dementia (FTD) often become apparent in fifty- or sixty-year-olds, making the disease relatively more common among younger people (see the Resources section at the back of this book for more recent information). Dr. Mesulam told us that PPA often seems to affect women in their sixties, like my mother. He didn't know why. He sounded more certain that she would soon lose almost all of her ability to speak.

"When?" we asked.

"Within a few years."

Mom said nothing, didn't sigh or make a sound as he continued. I sat behind her and couldn't see her face.

As the disease progressed, he told us, she would need help going to the bathroom, showering, dressing, and eat-

ing. We would see behavioral changes. And most likely dementia would spread throughout her brain. Eventually the
symptoms would resemble the last stage of AD. We learned
later that this meant she would probably disengage from
her environment, rarely say a word, and eventually lose
control of movement and the ability to swallow, among
other things. We waited for a shred of good news. But there
was none. The expert in front of us made it clear: there was
no known cure or even treatment for PPA.

I sat numb behind the rest of my family. I don't think my
mother shifted in her chair or moved a muscle during the
doctor's monologue. I don't know if she understood it.

Dad scribbled notes, as he had his entire career as a journalist. Writing was his defense, allowing him to distance
himself from a crisis while it was happening and make
sense of it later. He asked about medications. Mom already
had prescriptions for Namenda and Razadyne, two drugs
to heighten memory and awareness in Alzheimer's patients.
The doctor said she could keep taking them if there were
no negative side effects. There was no evidence that they
were effective against PPA, but his team was in the middle
of a study to find out. (Years later, he would report that Namenda didn't help people like my mother. It wasn't clear that
any other AD medications were effective, either; Mom had
tried one, Aricept, suffered stomachaches, and given it up.)

Without changing his clinical tone, the doctor addressed
two of the most emotional issues. "You should think about
retiring now," he told Mom. Soon her job would get to be

too difficult. The idea had already occurred to her, she said, her voice flat.

"And I am very concerned about your driving a car," he said. None of us nodded. We barely breathed. We knew that driving was an explosive issue between Mom and Dad. *Not today*, I thought. *Leave it alone for now.*

Jay helped to change the subject by asking whether the rest of us were at risk of inheriting PPA. It was a gutsy question. Over the previous few months, I'd worried every time I fumbled to find the right word or forgot the name of someone I'd met several times before. We braced ourselves for the answer.

"It doesn't appear to be inherited," Dr. Mesulam said. Later he and other researchers would report that specific gene mutations may in fact be linked to some cases, but no one else in our family had ever been stricken by it as far as we knew.

I continued to yearn for some fresh hope for my mother, maybe a story about one patient who'd beaten the odds. It never came. There was nothing left, except the growing realization that now these doctors needed us. PPA was rare enough that my mom had become a valuable research subject. It was time for more testing. All of her wrong answers and mistakes, though painful for us, would be important data for Dr. Mesulam and his team.

He offered a brain-donation form for us to fill out. If Mom chose to allow an autopsy of her brain, researchers might find out more about what had happened to her and why. The analysis of diseased tissue might open new avenues for treatments or cures. His office would let us know the results of future studies. And we would get confirmation of her diagnosis—a final iron-clad opinion after her death. It was the smallest of consolations, and jarring particularly to Jay.

He told me later he'd recently visited a morgue as part of his paramedic training. After the doctor suggested brain donation, Jay pictured Mom there, imagined the room where pathologists performed autopsies. The thought sickened him. How would brain donation help Mom? It wouldn't. The suggestion seemed callous at the very time my mother needed every remaining synapse in her head. All of us knew we wouldn't be able to sign away her brain in the course of a day like this.

Mom said nothing and asked no questions. She was escorted away for further evaluation.

THE REST OF US CROWDED into another small room for a session with a social worker.

"Tell me about your marriage," she said to my father.

"I call her Scout," Dad said, and then he couldn't speak. Until then, I'd rarely seen my father really cry. He sensed that the three of us, behind him, were moved by his silence. He turned toward us and saw my tears. "You too?" he said. He turned back to the social worker.

"Scout's been a guide for me all my married life," he said. "She's led me through hard times. Showed me how to do things I couldn't have done alone."

Now I was crying harder. I thought about the baby inside me and realized for the first time that he or she wouldn't know my mother the way I'd known her. *How much time will this child have with her? What is our life going to be like without Mom?*

And then: *What is life going to be like* with *Mom?*

Our social worker said few words as the four of us talked freely for the first time about our fears and loss. How could we stay in touch more? How could we support our father? How could we plan for the future? The session was soon over, and we'd asked more questions than found answers. We were sent back to the waiting room before we were ready.

Mom emerged from another office and joined us. She was red-faced, shaking her head. "Awful," she said quietly. "Awful. Awful. Awful."

Dr. Sandra Weintraub, a professor of psychology, behavioral sciences, and neurology at Feinberg, was by her side. She didn't volunteer any explanation for Mom's sadness. Later, after reading a clinical report of the results, we saw that my mother had given up in the middle of a test Dr. Weintraub administered. The doctor let us have a moment alone.

"Do you want to leave?" Dad asked. It would be easy to slip away because it was time for lunch. Each nod of her head spoke louder than words. *Yes. Hell yes.*

We ushered her into the elevator.

"Going down," a robotic female voice said after we pressed the button for the street level. When the doors opened, Mom took one step out into the lobby and began sobbing. Her body shuddered and she couldn't move her feet. We wrapped our arms around her in a tight bundle. We stood right there in the lobby instead of hustling her off to a private place where no one would see her breakdown. No more charades.

IT WAS TIME TO DECIDE whether we would return to the doctor's office for more tests that afternoon. We went to the first restaurant we saw, and quickly realized we were out of place. The crisp white tablecloths accented with delicate bud vases would've been just right for a birthday or anniversary. We were morose.

My mother didn't want to go back. We convinced her to endure one last scheduled session with Dr. Weintraub to see if she could give us any further advice. If nothing else, maybe Mom could register a complaint. She needed to vent her anger and sadness about the diagnosis and the debilitating way she'd learned the latest bad news.

We held her hands on the street and encouraged her to take deep breaths. I don't remember smelling any more chocolate in the air.

. . .

THE TESTING HAD TO END. We made that clear in the first thirty seconds after returning to Dr. Weintraub's office. I know she was disappointed to be losing a research subject, but she took our decision gracefully. I was proud that my mother was able to stand up for herself.

"And I never," Mom said, shaking her head and pointing in the direction of the door, "want that . . . other man."

"She doesn't want to see Dr. Mesulam again," Dad clarified. He was no doubt a brilliant doctor and scientist. My father learned later that he also had a big heart and a warm smile. It must have been hard for him to see our pain when he was delivering his diagnosis. But Mom elaborated.

"Awful," she said. "He . . . is . . . *terrible.*" The four of us nodded in support.

"That man," Dr. Weintraub told us quietly, "is my husband."

Oooh. We laughed awkwardly. *Sorry . . .*

This was a shocking moment of levity in the midst of a hard day, and Dr. Weintraub handled it with grace. Perhaps she'd heard the same feedback from others whose expectations had died on this floor. We asked more about the challenges we'd face in the coming years. She couldn't impart much new information. But she confirmed that my mother would need help with everything, and she recommended medication for her sadness. Mom was already taking Wellbutrin, with no side effects, for depression. Dr. Weintraub suggested switching to Paxil or Effexor, generally more effective for PPA patients. Apparently, Dr. Mesulam left issues about their patients' moods to his wife. She also recommended that Mom start speech therapy. Some evidence indicated that it might help temporarily.

Finally we raised one of the most sensitive questions relatives ask, about life expectancy. Dr. Weintraub wouldn't answer the question outright. It varies greatly from person to person, she said. We heard elsewhere that the longest any PPA patient had survived after diagnosis was nineteen years.

"What should I do?" Mom asked her. Her first question.

"Go home and be a grandmother," Dr. Weintraub said.

I thought, *How will she even do that?*

My mother was nervous as she sat at a glass table in front of an all-glass wall facing the beach. She and her friend and colleague Veronique, whom Mom called "V," had been invited into an immaculate house in Santa Monica, the home of a man with Parkinson's. They were there to share the latest information coming out of the foundation and to ask for a larger donation than the couple had previously given. His wife had led them into a large room with a marble staircase and a high ceiling, and told them her husband wasn't feeling well but that she'd love to hear what they had to say.

Following a plan built to Mom's strengths, V was to speak first in the meeting, outlining the latest news about research to find a cure for Parkinson's. Though Mom had trouble understanding the scientific material by then, she'd become very good at reaching for what her colleagues called "transforming gifts," dollar amounts higher than the comfort zone of the donor.

I can imagine that she felt exposed, fearing that V and the wife were watching her closely, maybe listening for mistakes or judging her. She had been told weeks earlier in Chicago that she would soon lose most of her ability to speak. Now she dreaded the loss of a few important words, the ones asking for more than this very generous couple had ever given before. She didn't want to come off looking unprofessional or unprepared.

My mother had made it clear that only family members and one or two close friends were to know what we'd learned during our traumatic time in Chicago. But just weeks after she and Dad got home, she revealed her diagnosis to the Fox Foundation, a group that had become a second family to her. Without drama, she told them why she'd have to retire at the end of 2006.

Her co-workers were startled and saddened by her admission that she was struggling to use the very fundraising skills she'd taught them. Those who'd been disappointed with her job performance over the previous months embraced her—and worried about her future. But Mom seemed resilient and wasn't much open to sympathy.

She publicly buried her sense of dread about her condition and aimed for even higher gifts for the foundation. It was especially bold of her to take this final fundraising trip to California in November. What did she have to lose? She wanted to go out with a bang.

In Santa Monica, V delivered her research report with ease. Then, before Mom could make her appeal, the woman's husband felt well enough to join them. In an instant the conversation warmed. His presence alone had leveled the playing field for my mother, as she realized that both of them struggled on the same team. This might have been my mother's moment to be honest with the couple about her own illness, but she wasn't ready to do that. Nevertheless, she seemed to be inspired and empowered by his presence, feeling a glow of mutually held goals.

She settled into her own playbook. She looked into their eyes. Thanked them for all they had done to support research.

She said, "We hope that you will consider doing something very special this year by increasing your support and making a gift of–"

She froze, silent. Nobody moved. I wonder what the couple must have thought. *Is she coming up with this figure on the spot? Is she afraid to ask? Is she hiding something?*

She tried again, rephrasing the question, but again when she got to the dollar amount the crucial words hid from her. She started humming. Sometimes this nudged her memory.

"Ahmmmmmm." The man and his wife looked uncomfortable. Finally Mom spoke.

"Twenty-five thousand dollars," she blurted out. She looked unprepared. Unsure. The couple might not have agreed to the donation if she had presented it perfectly, but they certainly weren't going to now. It was the man who let them know it wasn't going to happen this time. My mother knew she had missed her shot. She and V ended the meeting as quickly as they could and walked to the rental car.

There, freed from a fishbowl of observation, Mom started giggling. V had yearned for a happy ending to the appointment, but she knew what my mother needed now. They laughed from their bellies, burying their disappointment and dispelling the remnants of Mom's nervousness.

My mother lost that round, but not long afterward she won another. Remarkably, she was able to bring home one last donation for $2 million, one of the biggest gifts the foundation had so far received, and the largest amount ever given by a family that didn't have a personal connection to the disease. Her colleagues attributed much of that success to Mom's personal connection with the donor. She got down on the floor and played with their four-year-old son. She laughed easily and often during their time together and displayed an obvious passion for her cause. She didn't need words to make The Ask and land the gift.

Weeks later in December, as the New York City streets sparkled with colorful lights and holiday glitter, Mom knew it was time to go.

It was surreal and strange to her colleagues that she was

leaving. My mother worked hard at her desk, determined to finish the job well, after almost everyone else had left for the night.

IN EARLY 2007, ASHLEY THREW a surprise party in New York. It was meant to honor both of my parents' retirements, but my sister had a bigger plan in mind. She had written a dinner speech recapping Mom's diagnosis, projecting tough challenges in the years ahead, and asking for help from close friends. In a way, she was mirroring the process for fundraising work—not the standard agenda for a festive celebration.

All the fifteen or so guests knew about my mother's dementia after weeks of hushed individual briefings from Mom and Dad. They were all close family friends who had known us for years. The talks about the illness were always uncomfortable and usually ended with not-so-subtle pleas for privacy, like "We're not telling the world about this." Now my sister was ready to deliver an outspoken message, aimed particularly at Mom: We would no longer hold secrets, but we were there to support and love her.

I was getting close to the end of my pregnancy in Tennessee and couldn't travel. I hated not to be able to go but was there in spirit.

One of my mother's best friends, Anna, took a video of the evening, so I was able to watch it later. It captured the frenetic but loving energy Mom radiated at the time. It revealed some of the early symptoms of her disease. It also heightened my love and appreciation for my sister.

The recording is grainy, and the colors are dull in the evening glow of our dear friends Sheelah and Bill's house. Mom brightened the room when she arrived and shrieked, realizing that most of her favorite people had gathered to surprise her. She pointed at the camera with both hands. My dad stood next to her with his mouth open. He hadn't known about the party, either. My mother yelped to see each new person, covering her mouth, laughing. She noticed Veronique across the room and screamed louder than ever, rushing to hug her. Mom's childish giddiness overrode any nerves she might have felt about her then-constant struggle to find the right words.

"I am absolutely floored!" she said, looking around at her best friends.

"You had no idea?" Sheelah asked.

"I . . . nah . . . *no*!" Mom stuttered. "I can't believe that!"

She should have said, "I can't believe *this*"—a small difference that probably went overlooked at the time. But she often flubbed single words, disrupting her sentences with a kind of static.

"I just love that!" she said, looking around at the party and bouncing up and down. She rushed at the camera and hugged Anna, turning the frame sideways for a moment and showing a glimpse of Veronique's brown shoes. She walked into one of the dozen or more white ribbons dangling from helium balloons on the ceiling and didn't seem to realize what was brushing against the side of her face, but she saw an opportunity for a comic bit. She put her hands on her hips, smirking at the camera.

"What are you doing?" she asked, her face deadpan for a second, the string tickling her mouth as she talked. There was laughter from off camera.

"It's Ashley!" Mom yelled, grabbing my father's arm again, meaning, *This surprise party was thrown by Ashley.*

"I know," Dad answered. The story had been told several times in the span of a couple of minutes.

The party moved to a cozy dining room barely large enough to accommodate everyone. Tall candles lit the two long tables covered with wineglasses and generous servings of casseroles, potatoes, and cooked vegetables. V sat next to my dad, and Mom sat several seats away, laughing in the center of the packed and boisterous group, exactly where she liked to be.

My father stood up to make a toast.

"I was just thinking," he said, "how remarkable my life has become."

Someone giggled.

"Oh, *what*?" Dad said in mock anger. Uproarious laughter again.

"I feel," he continued, "I am Gurney in Wonderland tonight. And Linda is Alice, and we together have fallen down a hole to this remarkable place . . ."

A nice metaphor, typical of my father, and perhaps somewhat rosier than what had actually happened. My sister, sitting a couple of feet behind Mom, smiled as her eyes darted back and forth between both my parents.

There. A bit of truth. I could see the weight Ashley was carrying, and the burden we all felt those days anytime we were in a room with my mother. Ashley was trying to gauge, *Is Mom okay with this? Is she really happy? Or is she on the verge of breaking down?* My sister had become like a mother taking care of a young child, trying to foresee the fall that could come before the toddler gets to the top of the stairs. Ash was vigilant.

My dad's toast continued. ". . . thinking that we're falling into this pool of tears," he said, acknowledging for the first time why they were all gathered. Ashley's lips quivered, and her eyes squeezed shut for a moment. Again, I could see the truth as I watched it later: this was hard. I wanted to reach out and hug her.

"And instead," my dad continued, "we are surrounded by the waters of life and wine . . . and friendship and a rabbit saying, 'It's not late at all. . . .' Thank God for you all." People applauded. It was a sweet speech, and vague enough to acknowledge what was happening without really dealing with it. Mom mumbled something about how she didn't want to have to stand up and speak next. Others started teasing her, challenging her—maybe even to sing. No one expected her to, and she knew it. This was the kind of treatment she relished, honoring her, yet letting her off the hook from performing when she no longer could.

Minutes later my sister stood in front of the group, laptop in hand—she hadn't had time to print out her speech amid preparations for the party—and began reading from its screen.

"I am a lot like my mom," she said. "And I say that with swollen pride.... She's taught me how to embrace people, ideas, books, food, the beach—the things I love." My sister went on to describe the many disorganized traits they shared, like their inability to remember to close cabinet doors or pick up dirty socks off the floor. Her audience hooted and cheered.

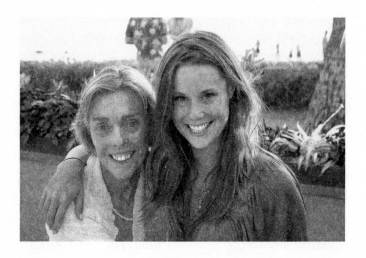

"You see," Ash continued, "at our cores, my mom and I are fascinated. We are dreamers. Creators. Builders. That means that when she is cleaning, she sees things and she can't help but stop and read. Hours later, she's dug through stacks and spread them out and is"—Ashley did an impres-

sion of Mom speaking with great pride—"working on a
project."

"That is completely true!" Mom yelled.

Next Ash listed the various ways my mom had been a
great fundraiser, and after every declaration, the group in
the room chorused, "Yes!"

"So," said Ash, taking a deep breath and slowing down,
"I wanna talk to you about something. Be here with me
right now. My mom is having tr—" Her voice cracked.

I heard my mother gasp. "Oh!"

The elephant. The truth.

"It's okay," Ashley said, pointing to her. "It's totally
good." The energy in the room shifted abruptly. Finally.

"'Cause we're happy and we're laughing. But there's
something we need to talk about." She took a breath. "It's
good," she added again, as if perhaps to convince both herself and Mom. *Here we begin a healthy dialogue.*

"Oh," my mother said again quietly. There was dread in
this moment, I'm sure, but also relief and resignation—for
my mother, and for the people who loved her.

Ashley continued: "My mom is having trouble finding
words."

It was the sentence all of us had wanted to say in public
on Mom's behalf for more than a year but hadn't yet been
allowed to. Nobody moved.

"She is slowly losing some of her brain function," she
continued. "And in many ways it's the part of her brain that
organizes things. The part of her brain that knows that she's

supposed to pick things up after herself, close the door behind her. . . . Between us, it's the part of both of our brains that's always sort of wanted a day off."

Big cathartic laugh from everyone.

"Yes!" Anna cheered.

"I think both of us are often overwhelmed by the exhaustion of keeping up with logistics: how things work, numbers, maps, schedules, time. Because—do you all realize? My mom and I are wonderers. Marvelers, wishers . . .

"Now, we don't know how this sickness is going to go. How fast, how hard. It is time for my mom to *play*." Big applause. Ashley was crying. Others dabbed their eyes. I couldn't see my mother.

"It's time for her to feel safe enough to dream, hope, stare, build, wonder, and feel surrounded by people who will respect her no matter what she does, laugh with her no matter how ridiculous." My sister looked directly toward Mom.

"I want you to feel free, Mom. Leave the cabinets open. Hug people as hard as you want to. Laugh loudly. Build big. Sleep heavy, walk lightly, and start making more messes in your brand-new kitchen. I think I speak for everyone when I say, *Go for it*. Follow your passion. And we will be here, applauding you at every turn. Call us. Have dinner with us, go for walks with us, paint us pictures, dance with us. We are your net, your blanket, your music, and your teammates."

The people in the room shouted approval when my sister finished her beautiful speech. She knew how to lay the truth out in front of this supportive group waiting to follow our family's lead. Ashley has a knack for that.

Then she presented Mom with a special gift.

My brother and sister and I had all received a "parachute book" from our parents when we left for college. Mom and Dad gathered up good report cards, kind letters, college recommendations, and our best papers, and pasted them in a book meant to encourage us when we needed it on our journey. To help us remember where we came from, what we've accomplished, and who loves us.

"So I have contacted everybody," my sister told my mom, "and everybody has written you something that is now in this book. And this is *your* parachute book. This is your parachute."

"Oh, Ash," my mother said, rising. They hugged and wept together for a brief moment. And then Mom flipped the mood.

"I wanna see it," she said dryly, grabbing the book off the table, relishing the laugh she knew she'd get. She didn't want to cry anymore. In that moment, Mom wanted to celebrate and feel the love surrounding her.

A FEW MINUTES LATER, FAMILY and friends gathered in the kitchen for cake. My mother picked up the knife and started to cut before blowing out the candles.

"Wait! What are you doing?" Ash said.

"Whoop!" Mom yelled.

"I think you're supposed to blow it out first."

"Wait a minute," Mom said, tapping her head and reaching her arms out toward the group. "What am I supposed to do?"

"Blow it out!" the friends cheered. She did, spitting a little on the cake.

Dad helped, huffing with her. Even though everyone there knew the truth now, both my father and my sister were in heavy work mode to save Mom from social mistakes.

My parents gripped the knife together, preparing to cut the chocolate cake the way they had at their wedding reception forty years earlier. They lifted the knife like an ax and chopped into the soft frosting. The first assault on the dessert was funny. But then Mom hacked at the cake again, threatening to butcher it. When she started for a third blow, Dad wrenched the blade from her, put a hand on her shoulder, and gently shook his head. Mom shrugged, palms up, as if to say, *What's his problem?*

"Food fight!" someone yelled. I wondered what they were all really thinking. They acted amused, loving, forgiving.

"Gimme that thing!" Sheelah said finally, smiling. She disarmed my parents and cut them two mauled slices.

"You guys gonna feed each other or what?" my sister said. Egged on by the group, Mom grabbed an entire piece of cake and slapped it onto Dad's face. It covered his mouth and chin for an instant before it fell off onto the floor. Mom won shrieks of approval for her audacity. Again, her comedic timing was good, but she teetered toward inappropriate. Dad pretended to shove a little piece of cake into her mouth. But her lips were closed and more clumps dropped to the floor.

The party was soon over. But not before Mom grabbed a fistful of chocolate and reared back, threatening to throw it at my father. Ashley jumped in front of him, holding her arms out to protect him.

It was an instinct Ash and all of the rest of us would have again soon. Things were about to get messy.

My mother's question hung in the air, day after day.
"*Where's the . . . ?*"

It was impossible to answer because she never completed it. And the silence filled my father with dread because it was a sign of the worst kind of loss. They could find or replace a purse or a pair of glasses. But he knew that my mother was on the verge of not even knowing what was gone.

Her illness had quickly become destructive, assaulting their marriage, putting their lives and the lives of others in danger. The battle in early 2007 was over driving. And the conflict was about to move to Tennessee.

After our son Huck was born in late February, I kept my parents at bay in New York for a few weeks so I could heal and focus on the whirlwind that was new parenthood. I wasn't allowed to go up and down stairs after having an epidural. I was sore, exhausted, and hungry all the time. I was trying to figure out the little insatiable creature who screamed for food and kept me up all night.

Brad loved being a father. He flew our son around the house, supporting Huck's tiny tummy on his forearm and his wobbly head and neck in the palm of his hand. They'd dart and turn, stop and hover in my face. Huck's eyes would open wide and he would coo at me, and then his dad would swing him away somewhere else. Brad let me pass out in the evening for a few hours after the last feeding (until the wee hours), rocking Huck back and forth to sleep in a Moses basket with that same strong arm.

My in-laws were a huge help, too. Sandy is the kind of woman who packs wet wipes, hand sanitizer, and the latest interesting-looking recipe clipped from *Good Housekeeping* in her purse. She can't walk into a kitchen without washing whatever is in the sink. She shopped, cleaned, and brought me a bowl of oatmeal in bed first thing each morning. Doug ran around fixing things and helped us set up the crib and changing table. The two of them are among the most energetic and generous people I have ever met.

My parents' arrival disrupted this serene household as if someone had dropped a beehive in our kitchen. Mom was furious because she wanted to drive Brad's oversized truck, as she had on previous visits. Dad argued that she wasn't in complete control of their old red Ford Explorer when she drove at home. She confused left and right, my dad said. She drove with one foot on the gas pedal and the other on the brake. She pumped the accelerator almost continuously, making the car lurch at an unsteady speed. My father told her he was afraid she would get hurt. She countered that he was too critical and cautious, the most irritating of backseat drivers. The part about him being irritating was probably true.

But we never talked about any of this while we were in the sunny living room of my house and the truck was parked outside on bright, springlike afternoons, as we gathered to stare at the new baby. Huck was our great distraction. Brad and I told my parents the story of the birth of their grandson over and over again. It was a kind of salve for Mom's wounded pride, and usually snapped her out of most bad moods.

Despite her disease, or perhaps because of it, she was a surprisingly charming and magical Nana (the nickname Huck would later invent), and I made sure to tell her so often.

"He loves you, see?" I said as Huck stared at her. He seemed fascinated as we lay on the floor with him and sang "You Are My Sunshine." My mother knew many of the words, and tapped the floor and hummed when she didn't. Huck loved the ruckus. He kicked and farted with glee.

Thank you, I told him in my mind. *For being delighted by us. And for having problems we can fix, like spit-up or a poopy diaper.*

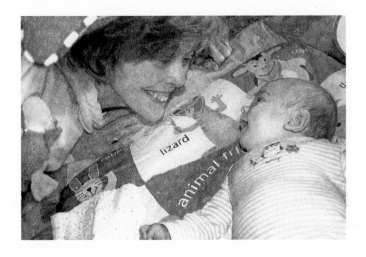

My mother held Huck awkwardly, but I never corrected her. And she never questioned or judged my maternal instincts. I was relieved not to suffer any of her criticism. She loved watching me become a mother, and the unsolicited advice she used to provide, the judgments about my choices, seemed to be gone. Her scrutiny of me had disappeared, replaced by an endearing show of humility and happiness.

I've often wondered what kind of grandmother she would have been without dementia. Maybe more reserved, more subdued. But as she was, she lay on the floor and cooed to my son much longer than I could before I ran out of energy. Her newfound playfulness evoked some of his first smiles. Her illness gave her a surprising gift: an intense joy that probably came from decreasing self-awareness.

. . .

BUT AWAY FROM THOSE SERENE scenes with me, Mom frequently shook with intense rage. My father downplayed to me his growing concerns about her driving, probably trying to minimize distractions from my role as new mom. I heard bits of the continuing story as I passed off Huck to him in the early dawn light of my kitchen while Mom slept.

Finally, exhausted, Dad gave up arguing about the car, chose marital peace over safety, and said she could do what she wanted. Curiously, after having won, Mom let him drive her everywhere for the rest of their trip.

But back home after the visit, she picked up the fight again. She often drove herself to Costco, a few miles from their house, and spent hours wandering up and down the giant aisles, stocking up on more than they needed—enough laundry soap, vitamin C, and toothpaste to last a year. When my father or anyone else offered to take her to the megastore and wait outside, she refused. I'm sure that driving there herself, pushing a large cart like other customers, and pausing to choose makeup or something Dad wouldn't know how to buy gave her a sense of competence.

But one day, inevitably, Mom confused the accelerator with the brake. The SUV barreled past a row of parked cars in the Costco lot and vaulted up the side of a two-foot-high retaining wall, coming to rest with its front wheels hanging above a hill on the other side. Remarkably, no one was hurt. The only damage was to the right rear fender of another vehicle. Its owner was kind and tried to comfort her. A tow truck hauled the car off the wall.

"I don't know what happened," my mom cried to the woman and a police officer at the scene. "I've never done anything like that in my life." That was true. The officer and the woman most likely wrote off any of her confusion after the accident as an emotional reaction to the wild ride. She walked away without consequence.

A few days later, Ashley arrived from California for a visit. She had no idea what had transpired when she offered to take Mom shopping—at Costco. My mother showed no fear of returning to the scene. Within seconds, as they pushed a cart past giant TV screens, a salesperson stopped them.

"How are you feeling, Mrs. Williams?" he asked.

How does he know Mom's name? my sister wondered.

"Oh, I'm fine," my mom mumbled, rolling by him.

"What's he talking about, Mom?" Ash said.

"Nothing," Mom said with a dismissive wave. "Stupid." It's possible she didn't remember all the details of what had happened. Even more likely, she didn't want anyone to know. Minutes later, another employee, looking concerned, asked the same question.

"Just silly," Mom said when Ash pressed.

When they got home, Ashley managed to corner Dad privately and force him to tell her the whole story. It was only because of her persistence that Jay and I heard about the incident. Mom had begged Dad not to tell us. We were very concerned that he'd agreed. It appeared as if even he believed the fiction that they were leading a normal life, or maybe her anger had just forced him to surrender and take her side. It felt premature and disrespectful to hide the keys from her, he told us later. Mom was still aware enough to see through any ruse. She was vulnerable and innocent, and he didn't want to hurt her.

We voiced our concerns to our parents, but Mom accused my siblings and me of "bashing" her about driving. She stopped talking to my father for a while, and then demanded that Dad stop talking to us about mistakes she made behind the wheel. So he stopped.

LATER THAT SUMMER, MOM AND Dad took a trip to New England with their friends Larry and Betsy. One day on the island of Nantucket, the group decided to rent bikes and follow the Polpis bike path, which ran a few miles east of the harbor. They found a shop that also offered motorbikes.

Dad's first hurdle was trying to convince Mom to go for the simple bike rather than motorized wheels. As a college student, she'd raced around the north of France with a boyfriend on a howling Harley motorcycle. Ever since, she'd yearned for the thrill of speeding in the open air. *What could go wrong with a little putt-putt scooter?* she wondered. The shop's staff told Mom she'd have to pass a brief driving test before she could operate the motorized bike, and she quickly dropped the idea.

They settled on ten-speeds, each with two brakes on the handlebars, one for the back wheel, the other for the front. They wore safety helmets. It was easy to put aside concerns about Mom's driving. *You never forget how to ride a bike,* Dad thought.

They set off sometime after lunch. My dad followed her as they left the town behind to make sure she was okay. Twenty minutes later, they started a long downhill, having pedaled hard to reach the top. My father passed her, probably saying something like "Lookin' good." He was relieved that she seemed to be in control. He shifted gears on the bike and felt the salt air in his face as he coasted. The sun was brilliant and the sky clear. When he got to the bottom, he realized my mother wasn't behind him. Then he heard her cry.

"Gurn! *Gurn!*"

He turned. Trees at the top of the hill blocked her from his sight.

"I'm coming, Scout!" he yelled. There were no other bikers around. Larry and Betsy were a few hundred yards behind him. Adrenaline propelled him back up the path.

He saw Mom on the ground, scared and sobbing.

"Scout," he said. "Oh, Scout." Blood covered her mouth, and the back of her hand was gashed. Dad tore off his T-shirt and wrapped the wound. She was missing a front tooth. He asked her if she felt pain anywhere else. "I don't know," she said. When their friends caught up, Betsy, a trained nurse, jumped off her bike and cradled Mom like a child.

"It was so scary," Mom cried over and over.

No one knows for sure what happened. But it seems likely that when she started down the hill, trying to keep up with Dad, she panicked at how fast she was moving. She probably yanked hard on the bike's front brake. It's the fastest way to stop. But the sudden deceleration can toss the rider headfirst over the handlebars. The helmet may have saved her life.

The ambulance arrived about fifteen minutes later on a road paralleling the bike path. Dad went with Mom to Nantucket Cottage Hospital. There she was taken away from him. A nurse gave Dad a green scrubs shirt to cover his naked torso and told him to stay in the waiting room.

But the staff soon learned that my mother couldn't tell them what happened. Her answer to every question was "Ask my husband." So they called my father in to help determine her "baseline." The challenge was trying to decide whether the accident had left her unable to communicate, or if her hesitation and confusion were always like this. Dad briefed the competent staff on PPA. They'd read about it but had never seen an actual case. Beyond their concern about possibly new neurological problems, the doctors were worried about Mom's complaint of abdominal pain—at least she was able to show them where she hurt—and the potential for internal injuries.

Larry and Betsy arrived at the hospital, bearing Mom's missing right front tooth with an intact root. Doctors implanted it, bandaged Mom's cuts, and kept her head and neck stable. But, still concerned about internal injuries, they decided that she needed to be helicoptered to Massachusetts General Hospital in Boston for testing and scans.

She was released the next day after spending a night there under observation.

Dad relayed the story to me over the phone from outside Mom's hospital room. I was sitting in my car in the CBS-Radford lot in Studio City, California, holding up a rehearsal for *According to Jim*. By that point, the cast had met my parents many times and knew what was going on with my mom. We were all gracious and patient with each other when a family issue like this came up for any of us.

The accident had been a blow to Mom's self-confidence, Dad said. It was another reminder that she couldn't be the adventurer she once was. That she needed assistance in things she used to do by herself. It was also yet another tug on his conscience, telling him that his wife shouldn't have been operating any kind of vehicle that moved faster than a walk. I was relieved to hear him say that. Three thousand miles away, I was overcommitted to work and to my growing family, and unable to fly home for long enough periods of time to really help. It was going to be up to my father to rein in our mom.

But even after her fall, she kept driving. Jay, Ashley, and I pointed out individually to Dad (because Mom still refused to discuss it with us) that she might kill someone—a child, perhaps, someone like her grandson. We pleaded for him not to let that happen. On top of that, we said, if Mom hurt or killed someone while she was behind the wheel, we would all be liable. He understood what we were saying and agreed, but still felt powerless. He didn't know how to stop her. He called the disease "the rat"—an intruder gnawing at her clarity, memory, and rational thinking. But it was becoming a presence in *his* head, too, frightening him, clouding his own reasoning. He let the rat rule.

And each of us, busy in other parts of the country, chose to say, "So be it." It was uncomfortable to question his judgment, and impossible to influence his decisions at a distance. I wish now I had fought my parents harder on it. I was learning as I went, and operating on a certain level of denial myself.

One day that summer, about a month after the bike accident, Mom's car ran out of gas after she'd driven herself to the beach close to their home. Unable to reach my dad, she started walking. A former high school classmate of mine, Sophie, found her by the side of the road and offered her a ride. It took a little coaxing to get Mom into the car. My friend's young child was screaming in the backseat.

Sophie didn't know that Mom had dementia. Few people did. "Where do you live now?" she asked. Mom's answer was jumbled and confusing.

My friend knew my parents had moved, but she didn't know where. She thought Mom was just being polite in not telling her where to go—as though my mother didn't want to burden her with having to take her home. She noticed a moment of clarity when Mom asked about Sophie's father, who was a doctor. Finally, though, with her little girl still yowling in the backseat, my friend deferred and let my mother out of the car by the side of the road. Both of them felt awful as they parted. Somehow my mother found her way home on foot.

The next day, Dad wrote out an apology for her on a piece of scrap paper. She rehearsed it over and over.

"I am sorry for the confusion yesterday. You were *very* kind to offer me a ride and I'm grateful." She bought a small potted plant as a thank-you gift, drove by herself to the right house, knocked on the door, and delivered her speech, cogent and clear.

In a rare move, my parents let me know what had happened. They said Mom was worried that she might be the subject of gossip. Grateful for permission to share the truth, I emailed Sophie right away, and for the first time told someone I didn't know very well anymore about my mother's sickness.

I wanted to thank you for helping my mom the other day.... She's dealing with a degenerative brain disease called primary progressive aphasia. It makes her confused and unable to speak sometimes, among other things. The disease is really rare, and we've just discovered she has it in the last year. I'm sure you noticed she was not totally herself.... If you see her again, I don't want you to feel like you should avoid her. It meant the world to her that you said hello and were so nice. ... I'm sorry if it was stressful or confusing for you.

She wrote back right away:

> Please emphasize to your mother that we all continue to hold her in high regard, and that the dignity with which she is obviously facing this challenge only serves to increase our respect for her.

I will always be grateful to Sophie for such an elegant response. It was exactly what I would have hoped for: that people wouldn't ostracize us because of Mom's illness.

FINALLY, AND FORTUNATELY, THE FORD Explorer got old. Dad exaggerated its mechanical failures and grumbled that it wasn't safe, hoping that Mom would agree they needed to trade it in. They both got excited about the idea of a cute little Prius. It was fuel-efficient and had a navigation system with a pleasant woman's voice that gave them directions.

Best of all, my dad secretly suspected that Mom wouldn't be able to figure out how to drive it, with its small and un-familiar "RNDB" control knob in lieu of a gearshift. The en-gine wouldn't start unless she pushed on the brake pedal at the same time she pressed a button on the dashboard—an engineering touch that Dad thought might keep her off the roads.

She insisted she wanted to practice in the new vehicle so she could learn to drive it. The conflicts got more and more intense. It was one of the hardest times for my father.

Belatedly, he offered to enlist the help of professionals. He told Mom that if she passed a formal driving test, then he would say he was sorry and agree he'd been too critical and cautious. Problem solved.

Giving her false hope was an antidote to further poisonous fights. And she was finally off the roads. But it meant that now he (and others) had to participate in a series of pretend training sessions in a large and usually empty parking lot near their home where all three of us kids had learned to drive.

As he worked with her throughout the summer of 2008, he suffered stomachaches whenever they got to the parking lot. With his help, Mom was able to make the car go forward and back, but she had trouble following directions like "Take us toward the light post."

Their preparations for the test—one that everyone but Mom knew would never happen—stretched into the fall and winter.

"How is the Prius?" I asked on the phone, in a vague way trying to encourage her to talk about driving.

"Great!" was all she would say.

One weekend Ashley flew home and offered to be Mom's instructor for an afternoon, as she'd done often. She took Mom in the Prius to the empty lot. They stopped and traded seats.

"What's the very first thing you need to do when you get into any car?" Ash asked. Mom tapped the dash, adjusted the mirror, and slapped the wheel, but she didn't know rule number one: *Fasten your seat belt.* She never got close to starting the car.

"I'm never gonna get this, am I?" she said finally.

Ashley turned to face our mother.

"No, I don't think so, Mom," she said.

"I've lost my . . ." Mom paused to find the word. "Authorship."

My sister gasped. Somehow, in her jumbled brain, my mother had found a word close to "autonomy," and in the moment, it perfectly described what she'd lost. Ashley burst into tears.

"Oh!" Mom said, and wrapped her arms around my sister, comforting her.

"It's not safe for you to drive, Mom," Ash said, weeping.

She felt my mom's chest shudder, and then, in another moment of clarity, Mom finally answered, "I know."

SHE NEVER DROVE AGAIN, THOUGH sometimes she forgot why she couldn't. Within months, even her desire to try faded away.

A quirky collection of vehicles lined up at the edge of our pond in the late spring of 2008, like preparations for some kind of parade. The music—"Surfin' Safari"—blared from speakers in Brad's truck. Its blue hood gleamed in the sun. Squatting next to it was our yellow skid-steer loader, a slow-moving machine the size of a baby elephant, which Brad and Huck (in a baby carrier) would ride for joyful hours at a time, moving small boulders from here to there.

My parents' silver Prius hybrid, a clown car by comparison, had brought Mom and Dad from New York. And my self-proclaimed "redneck relatives," the Getzelmanns, had poured out of their overstuffed red minivan when they'd arrived from North Carolina.

The family gathering was an ambitious Brad production, blending southern farm and northern suburb, toddlers and newlyweds, parents and grandparents all together in a mixture of circus and sitcom. My husband had loved having the extended family together for Christmas months earlier, and had particularly bonded with my cousin Stephen over being a new dad.

Brad wanted to get the whole group together again for a silly reunion. It would be the two of us, Huck, Holler, Ash, Aunt Diana (Mom's sister), Uncle Bill, Stephen and his wife, Beth, their newly adopted son, Tyler, Jay and his wife, Adrienne, Sandy and Doug, and my mom and dad. My in-laws had recently moved nearby. So had my brother and his wife. Everyone else would stay on the property. We'd converted the old farmhouse into a studio and guesthouse, and built a log cabin in the woods, where we now lived. Our guests would crash wherever they could—in guest bedrooms, on couches and floors—for three nights.

Brad's plan was derived from a 1997 *Seinfeld* episode that introduced the world to a fictional holiday called Festivus. It was based on an actual family tradition for one of the show's writers, Dan O'Keefe. In his version, the rampant commercialization of Christmas destroys peace and goodwill among men. Two of the characters actually come to blows over the last doll in a store. One of them, George Costanza's father (played by Jerry Stiller), realizes there has to be a better way. In O'Keefe's script, the celebration begins when you gather your family around "and tell them all the ways they have disappointed you over the past year." It was one of Brad's favorite episodes.

Our Festivus would be a slightly friendlier version. It would be the opposite of stuffy, and the only pressure we'd put on one another would be to keep a sense of humor and do whatever we wanted to do. It would be the antidote to all of the ghosts of Christmases past. Out of necessity, but best of all, the ringleader in many ways would be my mother. We would follow her recent lead in throwing etiquette out the window.

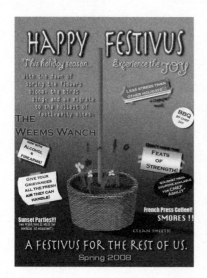

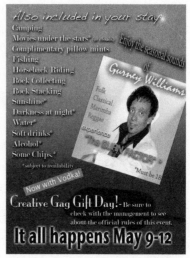

MY HUSBAND'S GARISH, HASTILY MADE invitation promised the main events and features of *Seinfeld*'s Festivus. His full-color Photoshopped digital creation made it clear that it was an unholy holiday. Instead of a tree, we'd set up a bare aluminum pole. Instead of presents, we'd have a gag gift exchange, a way to get rid of old stuff we didn't want. There would be "Feats of Strength" (haphazard dinghy races across the pond for the prize of the Festivus Dixie Cup), "Sunset Parties (so wild you'll still be rockin' at sunrise)," and, lastly, "some chips (subject to availability)."

Everyone accepted the invitation with great enthusiasm. Ashley volunteered to take on the role of Director of Schedules and Activities, with events including an "Airing of Grievances," fishing, napping, and drinking beer whenever we wanted. Jay and Adrienne offered to cook ribs on the grill. The Getzelmanns planned to make their famous seven-layer Mexican dip. Mom and Dad practiced a special performance. I put together "gifts" for each person, filling used paper or plastic bags with things like expired Emergen-C powder, stale gum, Band-Aids, and half-used packages of Alka-Seltzer. Brad made a special playlist including songs from the Beach Boys, Hank Williams Jr., Jimmy Buffett, and Andy Griffith. We bought the ingredients for s'mores, bottles of bug spray and beer, and tubes of sunscreen. After briefly looking around the farm for an aluminum pole, we settled instead on a broken broomstick.

Once everyone arrived, the party began. We congregated at the edge of the pond on a twenty-foot-long stretch of sand Brad and Huck had created with the skid-steer. We called it Betty Beach, named after my grandmother. I walked around with a video camera, documenting. While Brad worked the soundtrack ("Cheeseburger in Paradise" came up after "Surfin' Safari"), Doug and Uncle Bill gathered fishing gear and Stephen helped Tyler, age two, catch his first bluegill.

"That would be a party foul," my cousin said with a smirk, holding up a broken fishing pole. "You do not break the rod while catching the smallest fish of the day."

"Grievance!" I shouted.

"Good news," he added, his blue eyes sparkling, "is that Tyler got his first fish."

Mom, Diana, Beth, and Sandy danced the Twist next to the remnants of seven-layer dip and a half-eaten bag of stale chips.

"Woo!" my mother yelled, arms swinging. Gone were many of her feelings of propriety. And in some ways, she seemed the happiest she'd ever been. She adored everyone and everything. She treasured having the family together. She loved being a grandmother. She'd always been quick to laugh around Diana. Years before, when Stephen and I were kids, we'd watch the two sisters as they raced lobsters across the floor or cackled over some fantastic secret we weren't supposed to know. At Festivus, despite the obvious progression of PPA, Mom giggled with Aunt Di as much as ever.

"Sand!" she cheered to one-year-old Huck when he face-planted and ate a mouthful of it for the first time. Her shorter responses were ideal for communication with a toddler, and to him she seemed not only perfectly normal but really fun.

Dad was the only one who was suffering. He looked tired, despite putting up a front. I'm sure he was dealing with a lot more struggles than we knew, but he was good at hiding many of them from us. As always, Mom wanted him to keep the real challenges private.

He and I each pulled two small metal boats into the water to race for the only scheduled "Feat of Strength." My partner, Sandy, dutifully sat behind me as I paddled us both across the one-and-a-half-acre pond.

"Come on, Kimmy! You can do better than that!" Aunt Diana chided from shore.

Mom sat in the back of the other boat with Dad, slapping and pushing on his shoulders as though that would increase his speed.

"Go, Gurn, go!" she howled. "Fast!"

Though she was enjoying herself, Mom knew less and less about what was going on—how to follow conversations, how to use an oar. But it didn't seem to bother her much, and she made up in enthusiasm what she lacked in understanding. Brad videotaped us from the shore and tried to shout directions, to no avail. Stephen snorted and kept on fishing. Mom and Dad won the race, and my father pumped his paddle in the air. Everyone cheered. Dad maneuvered to shore and got out of the boat. From behind the camera, Brad asked him how he felt.

"It was a generational race," my dad said. "Younger people are a lot worse than older people." They heard Mom cackle.

"Gurn!" she shouted, and giggled again. She was still in the dinghy, uncertain about how to disembark. Dad ran back to her and used both hands to pull her up out of the wobbly boat. He barely avoided soaking them both in pond water.

We cleaned up slightly and met for cocktail hour on our deck overlooking the farm. I was inside when I heard my mother's shriek of surprise. She had accidentally walked into the closed screen door from the porch, knocking it off its hinges. It clattered sideways, but no one was hurt (although the door never closed straight again). It only briefly stopped the party. We helped her laugh it off.

Brad timed a different playlist to the setting of the sun, culminating with the theme song from *2001: A Space Odyssey*, "Thus Spake Zarathustra." We put arms around each other, watched the last rays disappear behind the hills, and toasted to a grand, irreverent day.

It was then that Mom dropped a glass. She must have gotten distracted or confused. I heard it shatter on the porch. We put shoes on Huck and Tyler, whisking them away from the mess, and cleaned up the shards with a dustpan and broom in the dimming light. Mom was apologetic and embarrassed, but again we laughed and reassured her. We replaced her drink and said it was no big deal. When she broke her second glass, we switched everyone to plastic so my mother wouldn't feel singled out.

Later that evening, we all sat around the table for dinner, and the "Airing of Grievances" never got more insulting than "Your socks have holes in them" or "You double-dipped your chip." The few jokes about breaking down screen doors or smashing glasses were good-natured. Mom didn't stop smiling.

I'll never forget the final night of what everyone agreed was a successful first annual Festivus. We'd just finished dinner. Sandy held Huck, who cooed and pointed. Tyler shuffled around his mother's feet. Stephen stood watching from behind his handheld camera, which he used to record almost everything. Aunt Diana was cackling even before the evening's entertainment began.

My parents were preparing to perform a musical finale. Dad's expression was mock-serious, but it was hard not to smile at his half of the orchestra. It was a kazoo, crafted out of a long leafy twig from our woods. He had slit open one end of this instrument and jammed a tiny paper reed into the crack. Mom stood next to him. She was the other half of the ensemble, the entire percussion and giggles section, holding a pair of stew-pot lids.

"We will now perform for you the final movement of Beethoven's Ninth Symphony in D Minor," Dad announced, and cleared his throat.

In its original form, the movement was the choral climax of one of the most popular classical pieces in the world, with words from Friedrich Schiller's poem "Ode to Joy." Recently I looked up the English translation of the words, none of which were sung in my parents' truncated rendition. What went unspoken strikes me as poignant now.

Joy is the name of the strong spring
in eternal nature . . .
Joy drives the wheels in the great clock of worlds . . .

The happiness we felt, possibly romanticized in my memory, still feeds me years later. The evening was one of the last times we'd all be together. In the next couple of years, our larger family would change dramatically, in predictable ways and also in unexpected ones. But in that moment, huddled in our country kitchen, all was well. We snickered as Dad raised the twig to his lips and blew. The kazoo squealed in time and on pitch (as far as I knew). At the end of every couple of bars he turned to Mom, who stood next to him expectantly.

Whoever has won a lovely woman—
Add in his jubilation!

Each time she got the nod from him, she raised her metal pot lids and banged them together. Kids jumped. Mom giggled.

Beethoven's Ninth has never been played as it was in the abridged version my parents performed that night. Dad ended on a high triumphant squeak, followed by Mom's final clang.

Close the holy circle tighter
Swear by this golden vine:

Remain true to the vows
A serene departing hour!

DAYS LATER, RAIN WASHED AWAY Betty Beach, and over the summer the water seeped out of the pond. We spent the next two years rebuilding it. We celebrated Festivus twice more after that weekend, but none would ever be as fun as the first.

We were a cheery crew during our irreverent celebration. My heart ached when the family dispersed and we reverted to our roles as long-distance caregivers. But we were grateful for the memories of the days together, especially the realization that my mother had become more accepting of her own shortcomings.

In the months that followed, she allowed my dad to print up a list of guidelines to help friends talk with her. The style resonated with the cheeky tone of Festivus, but the message drew on serious advice from the Burke Rehabilitation Center in White Plains, New York, where she was receiving speech therapy.

Dear smart, funny, sensitive, and supportive friends,
Conversation is the best speech therapy. Burke views

talking with Linda as a way to show what she knows, thinks, and feels. Conversation can reveal and acknowledge her competence, Burke says. Thinking about talking in this way has helped her. She is far more fluent and confident than she was before we got serious about Burke work.

Good things to do:
Provide extra time for Linda to process what you are saying and extra time to respond.
Keep explanations short and simple, but also adult.
Compound sentences (strings of ideas connected with conjunctions) compound communication difficulties and make it less likely she'll understand and make you appear boring and are not a great thing to do and sometimes make anybody forget what the beginning of the sentence was about.
Keep your voice at a normal volume. This may be impossible for this group.
Use gestures with the ease but not the extravagance of an Italian.

Not-so-good things to do:
Don't finish Linda's sentences or supply the word she's seeking unless she asks, often nonverbally by punching you, for help.
Don't interrupt. It can cause her to lose her place.
Don't be afraid of silences.

Don't limit conversation to activities of daily living,
although sex is fair game although daily sex is but a
dream and not necessarily her dream.

ASH FLEW TO MOM AND Dad in New York every month
or two from Los Angeles to cook meals, pick up around the
house, or take Mom to speech therapy appointments. These
occasional visits were frustrating for her. She noticed that
Dad wasn't delegating enough of the caregiving chores to
friends or hired help. She saw how much he was taking care
of our mother, and she was haunted by that lunch at La
Bonne Soupe and Mom's plea: *I don't ever want Daddy to
take care of me.* Ashley told my dad about the conversation,
but because my mother hadn't written her wishes down,
and because she had only said it to my sister, my father dismissed it. He didn't understand what his wife might have
meant. *She didn't want to be a burden? But what did she actually want me to do?*

He never had the courage to ask her. And our mother's
perspective had changed. She didn't want anyone helping
her *except* our father. Mom had forgotten the promise she'd
asked Ash to keep, and didn't realize how much Dad was
doing for her. In fact, he seemed to take great pride in being
the only one she wanted help from.

In between visits, my brother and I tried to reach out
over the miles separating us from New York. Jay created
a book with pictures—of people, places, and things—our

mother could point to when she couldn't retrieve a word. He sent it off but heard nothing back. I called home often. The sharpest pain for me was hearing Dad's voice straining to sound happy while Mom listened. All of us were living in shadows and half-truths about what was happening.

Then my father and I stumbled into a project that allowed us to connect outside of and apart from Mom's illness. We began writing a young adult novel about a secret army of intelligent farm animals led by a snake, patterned after the villain of Eden. The story was Dad's idea, and he asked me to develop it with him. I savored the opportunity. We found a literary agent in New York, and that allowed my father to classify the project as serious employment, requiring him to take time away from caregiving. For the first time in months, he and I could talk privately. Initially, at least, Mom left him alone during what we thought of as "office hours."

We wrote, edited, expanded, and revised more than thirty drafts of the book in 2008 alone. The fiction was less important for me than the opportunity to ask him about his real-life trials at home, though he never wanted to discuss them for long.

"I have to think of taking care of your mother as my new job," he told me. "If I do that, it's really not the worst I've ever had. I enjoy it." Even when he was trying to be honest with me, he was determined to sound sunny in the middle of a storm. The truth was, he told me only later, the job was so hard for him at times that he felt uncomfortable asking anyone else to take it on.

He tried to enlist her help in making dinners. She was earnest, stubborn, and sensitive—her disease hadn't robbed her of these endearing traits—and Dad had to coach her casually without offending her pride.

"What's the measuring cup doing next to the beans?" she asked.

"I forgot to tell you. All you have to do is fill it all the way up."

"Okay, but what do I do after I put them in the cup?"

He also tried to set up the house to give her more autonomous control over her life. He wrote out operating instructions for how to make coffee and how to push the auto-dial buttons on their landline. He stuck a Post-it note saying, "Press here" on the microwave keypad with an arrow pointing to "ADD 30 SEC" so she could heat up milk by herself.

But the note confused my mother.

"This?" she'd say, pressing the yellow slip instead of the shortcut key.

Dad couldn't imagine that anyone else would know Mom well enough to keep her from being hurt or even more discouraged than the disease already had made her. And that meant he was anchored to caregiving with little chance of arranging time off with friends, even though several of them and his therapist encouraged him, as my siblings and I did, to take better care of himself.

The range of communication between my parents had narrowed. His therapist suggested it was as if an entire piano keyboard had shrunk down to just four notes. My father thought he was the only one who knew how to play them.

The truth was that nobody could stop the onslaught of her disease. In speech therapy sessions at Burke, Mom was having trouble following even simple directions: "Make a fist and open your mouth." Or "Squeeze my hand and look up at the ceiling." Her therapist provided homework, like practice with writing numerals. One day my mother stared at the numbers she'd written, one to five.

"I don't get what they mean," she told my father. "I'm not sure what we're doing. I know this is three, this is four, but why is that?"

Her determination broke my heart. I tried to imagine what it must have felt like to be her. It was as if, for no apparent reason, the puzzle pieces that always used to fit to-

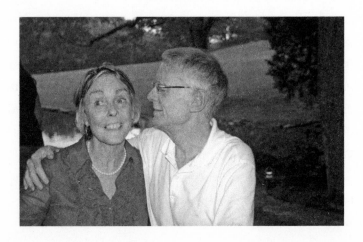

gether didn't anymore. Even the purpose of numbers didn't make sense. She blamed herself for not understanding. She thought that if she could just tough it out, try just a little harder, she could overcome the challenges of her daily life.

Jay said Mom's sickness felt like "death by paper cut"—tiny wounds of attrition with every new loss—and that's how it felt to me, too.

BUT THERE WERE STILL REASONS to celebrate. At the end of 2008, I got pregnant again. The second time around, it was fun telling my parents. All the fear I'd felt the first time was gone. Brad wrote a sign that said, *I'm going to be a big brother* and gave it to Huck to hold from his high chair. Then we Skyped with them and asked if they wanted to see their grandchild. When Huck held up the sign, my dad read it to Mom, and they both started cheering. My mother soon switched to screaming, in typical fashion, but she understood what was happening, and was ecstatic. Huck looked confused by her over-the-top reaction but was pleased to have caused such a ruckus.

This pregnancy flew by. As soon as my belly began to pop out, I coincidentally got offered a role as a guest star in the series finale of one of my favorite shows at the time, David E. Kelley's *Boston Legal*.

I hadn't been working much since having Huck. I wanted to focus on my family and being a mom, and faced with Brad's busy schedule, I felt that the time was right to take a break from acting. *According to Jim* had ended, and I'd started to get picky about taking on other projects. But this part seemed to have been written for me. The character I'd be playing, Hilary, the "wonder girl from Tennessee," was a lawyer arguing in front of the Supreme Court alongside my two favorite characters on the show, played by phenomenal actors William Shatner and James Spader. And to top it off, the argument in court was about an experimental drug for Alzheimer's. *Wow.*

At first I was concerned my newly bulging tummy would keep me from acting the role. Kelley assured me that it wouldn't be a problem: Lawyers get pregnant, too. My next challenge was memorizing pages of brilliant dialogue. I'd never had a problem learning lines before, but now I was paranoid.

Mom's disease was at the forefront of my mind, though I still hadn't discussed it publicly. Seeing her struggle to find words made me insecure every time I couldn't find one myself. *Am I showing early signs of PPA?* part of me wondered, and probably always will. But my actual condition was what is more commonly referred to among my friends as "mommy brain." I was pregnant and also caring for a toddler. I was exhausted, distracted, and emotionally drained. The neurons in my head accustomed to memorization were on vacation. My body was being taken over by a demanding little stowaway already stealing protein from my plate.

I was determined to succeed at this job and hold my own in court. I recited my speeches over and over to myself—

before bed, first thing in the morning, in the car, on the plane. I was careful to enunciate words like *scrupulous*, *efficacy*, and *permissive advertising* because I wanted to sound as if they were in my vocabulary every day (yeah, right—in between diaper changes and the sixth round of "The Itsy Bitsy Spider").

Hilary was arguing against letting Shatner's character, Denny Crane, who had Alzheimer's, take an unapproved drug despite the absence of clinical trials. In a scene in a bar the night before the trial, Crane sits down next to Hilary and says, "I have Alzheimer's disease." And Hilary says, "You're not alone. Over five million Americans do, including my own grandmother." For the first time, I was helping to raise awareness for the most common form of dementia, while only a small group of people knew my family was facing dementia at home.

The next day in our staged Supreme Court, I got through the bulk of my monologue with barely a stutter, and relished Spader's character's line when he leans over to his partner, Crane, and whispers, "She's *good*." (Career highlight—even if it was just a line in the script.)

And then Spader's monologue slayed me. He had always been funny and convincing as he spouted legal jargon. In the final round of the series, his character was arguing on behalf of someone he loved about a subject close to my heart.

"Denny has a sense of wonder and innocence like a child with all of the world before him," he says. "He has that capacity for sheer joy that most of us somehow lose along the road to adulthood.

"I love him with all my heart," he goes on. "My best friend is dying of an incurable disease that will rob him of himself before it finally robs him of his life." I choked up and fat tears rolled down my cheek every time we repeated the scene.

After one of the takes, the director, Bill D'Elia, asked me if I thought my character would really be crying in appreciation of an opposing counsel's argument when she has actually just lost.

I said, "This is hard for both sides. My mother actually has dementia. It's not easy, no matter which way you look at it." *There.* I'd said it. To someone I didn't even know. It just came out. And I didn't even say, *Don't tell anybody, but . . .* D'Elia listened and didn't respond. But he didn't freak out, either. *It doesn't have to be a big deal,* I realized. Everybody has stuff they're dealing with.

"I'll do one without crying," I said. "You can choose."

When the episode aired, they used one of the takes with the tears.

AT HOME, WE WERE BUSY moving Huck out of the nursery and making room for another child. I decided to use a midwife, and was planning on self-soothing during labor with hypnosis and a birthing tub newly installed at Vanderbilt University Medical Center. This baby's delivery was going to be *au naturel*. Mom had opted for drug-free births with all three kids. Why couldn't I do it for one?

So of course I wound up having to have a C-section. I wasn't aware that in the two weeks he spent past his due date in my womb, Jasper had grown to a formidable 9.2 pounds. He was in a bad position for delivery. And his heart rate was dropping too much during contractions. My mid-wife, Emma, was concerned enough to alert the doctor on call at the hospital. And he was anxious enough to run—perhaps sprint—to our room.

It alarmed me that he was out of breath when we met him, but Dr. Beyer delivered Jasper with great skill and kindness.

"He's smiling at me!" he said when he first saw my son's face looking up at him. I was behind a big blue screen, so I couldn't see anything. But Brad watched as the doctor held up the baby. I heard a slight gasp and a few chuckles.

"He's huge!" someone said.

The first thing *I* noticed was his dimples.

I asked my parents to wait a whole month before visiting from New York. I needed time to acclimate to juggling two children. And I had even less confidence than last time about Mom's ability to help, given her decline. Actually, it was more than that. I had real concerns for Jasper's safety.

My fears turned out to be warranted. Once my parents arrived, Mom insisted on holding him. That was fine with me as long as we were sitting together on the couch. I was always a stickler for hand washing. But when Mom forgot the soap, wet her hands a little, and wiped them on the butt of her pants, I let it slide. Thank goodness Jasper was the second child.

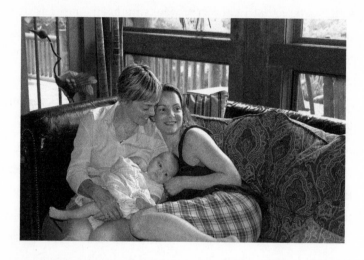

One day during my parents' visit, I was getting my hair and makeup done in the living room for an event that evening. Jasper was sleeping in his little Moses basket nearby, and Mom was hanging out with us. Dad had disappeared. I was happy to be allowing him a break. While chatting with Robin, the makeup artist, I hadn't noticed that Jasper had quietly awakened. So I was startled to see my mother carrying him in her arms.

Her grip was awkward. Jasper's blanket was askew, falling off in a long train toward the floor. She could easily have tripped over it. I wanted to hop out of the chair and snatch him away, but I was afraid to offend her. In that moment I made a conscious decision to let her be a grandma, in turn letting myself buy into the fantasy that just for a minute everything was normal.

Then I saw Jasper's head slipping out of my mother's arms as he arched backward. She caught his legs and was able to stop his fall a few inches before he hit the floor. She held him there by his feet, dangling upside down.

I gasped, jumped out of my chair, and grabbed him.

"Oh my God!" I exclaimed. I was furious, on the verge of yelling at her.

Her face flushed with embarrassment, and—to my surprise—anger at *me*. She was enraged that I had snatched the baby out of her arms, and humiliated by my reaction. *It was Jasper's fault, not mine,* she tried to tell me in broken sentences. As she continued rambling, I sensed how upset she was. I fought to stay calm.

"No big deal," I said.

But I was shaking and my heart was racing. I clutched Jasper tightly to me. As I walked back to my seat, I saw the horrified expression on Robin's face.

How could I have let that happen? I thought. Mom went into the bathroom, probably to cry. I turned to Robin and whispered, "Did you see that?"

"Yes!" she said, equally concerned. We were afraid to say anything else. Mom would be able to hear, and I already knew that my father and I would be dealing with her shame and fury for at least the rest of the day.

I didn't bring it up with Brad at the time. I didn't want to worry him. But it felt as if the ground had turned to slippery ice, and I was struggling to get my balance. I realized with certainty that my most important job was to protect my children from their failing grandmother, a challenge I had never expected to have.

What else could go wrong? My mind scrolled through as many disaster scenarios as I could imagine. What was once a safe cabin turned into a terrifying danger zone as my mind filled in the blanks. I imagined my babies tumbling from my mother's arms and down the stairs, off the balcony, or out a window. What if she tried to feed them Legos instead of peas? What if she picked them up by the neck? (That almost happened later, but I was there to stop her.)

Suddenly nothing was beyond the realm of possibility.

I realized that another adult and I would have to be home with my boys anytime my mother was there, in case of emergency. We would have to watch my mother and kids constantly, and know how to steer Mom away from potentially dangerous situations. Ideally, the double-team arrangement had to be set up discreetly to protect my mother from a catastrophic emotional crash if she found out about it. My mind spun out of control, wondering what else I could be missing.

My parents' departure could not have come soon enough.

BY THE MIDDLE OF THAT summer, we noticed Mom needed help eating food. Once it was on her plate, she usually ate with the wrong utensil. She tried using a spoon or a knife as a fork to eat long strands of spaghetti. Mealtimes were messier with Mom at the table than they were for my children. Like them, she often needed a change of clothes afterward. Extra napkins didn't help. She bunched them up to wipe her mouth and tossed them aside, leaving her lap wide open. I was embarrassed for her, but she didn't seem to mind the mess she was making. So, like many other things, we laughed it off and cleaned it up.

Eventually she wouldn't let my father work alone as often, so he and I weren't able to talk as easily. With Dad's increasing duties as 24/7 caregiver and mine as a new mother of two, the book project fell away. My father had always been thin. Now he was losing weight and appeared frail to us. He didn't have the focus that he'd once had. He called less and less often, and rarely responded to voice messages or emails. We went to New York whenever we could. But we couldn't be there all the time, so we were living in dread about what was happening to them at home.

Mom started meeting Dad's attempts to help with toxic resentment. Her face reddened, and she became sullen, distant, angry. She couldn't say how she felt, and hated him for not guessing correctly. They fought when she wanted to walk outside, by herself, in a storm. She wanted to experience the excitement as she always had, but no longer understood its potential dangers. She couldn't be left at home for fear she might hurt herself and not know how to get help. But most of the time she didn't want to be alone, and it was harder and harder for my dad to get even a little time to recharge.

All the same, he wondered how much grief he would feel when this intractable stubbornness began to fade. Now, though, it was too intense, like a lightbulb with blinding wattage.

In a rare move to get help for himself, he signed up for a caregivers symposium at Northwestern in August 2009. The Cognitive Neurology and Alzheimer's Disease Center had stayed in touch with him, keeping track of Mom from afar and sending my father updates on research and information on support groups. More than anything, he thought the event would be a legitimate reason to take some respite time. Our friend Anna volunteered to stay with Mom so Dad could get away.

At the conference, he learned more about the latest research on frontotemporal disorders, including PPA. He went to a support group meeting and without being asked took on the role of breaking the ice in the discussion, telling a little of his story and showing sympathy for other participants. He was surprised when the actual leader of the session, our old friend Dr. Weintraub, pulled him aside afterward. Maybe, he thought, she would thank him for helping her facilitate.

"Have you considered getting treatment for depression?" she asked. He hadn't. He was so focused on my mother's mental state and so out of touch with his own that it hadn't occurred to him that he'd shown any vulnerability or sadness.

Rather than being a relief, the conference ended up having the opposite effect on him: The brief distance had allowed him to see clearly that PPA was a horror, and it left him drained.

In sharing this new awareness with my mother in their living room afterward, he began by talking about all the positives in their lives—the kids and grandkids, the good works she'd done, her laughter and joy in life, his love for her. Then he hit her with the big news: He needed to get away more. He felt depleted. Depressed, he admitted. My mother cried quietly and said, "I'm sorry." He tried to get her to talk more about how she felt, but she couldn't add anything else.

He hired a woman from the local YMCA, Laura, whom Mom loved, to come once a week or so to take her out or just to do things with her at home, allowing Dad some quiet periods to be by himself. At first, she was happy with the arrangement. My brother and sister and I thought it was hardly enough, but our dad was adamant that he knew what they needed.

EARLY ONE MORNING THAT FALL, sitting at his desk downstairs at home, Dad noticed an uncomfortable tightness in his chest. He started sweating and became nauseated and short of breath. His parents had both died of cardiovascular disease, and my dad had spent years later editing a newsletter, the *Cleveland Clinic Heart Advisor*. So he was familiar with these four signs of a heart attack and knew they should be taken seriously. He didn't want to be the medical journalist who'd instructed readers when to call for help but then ignored his own advice.

Mom, having just woken up, appeared at the door of his office. *This is really going to be hard for Linda* was Dad's first thought. He knew he needed to take a potentially life-saving step without scaring her.

"Scout," he said, "I'm so sorry. Things are about to get a little chaotic. I'm going to have to call 911."

"Oh! Oh! Oh!" Mom grabbed at his arms.

"I'm gonna be fine," he went on. "I'm just feeling some symptoms in my chest that I've written about." Again he said, "I'm so sorry."

He dialed 911 from his office phone. Mom was pacing, anxious.

"Why don't you go get dressed? You'll come with me to the hospital."

"Okay!" my mother said, and ran upstairs.

Dad lay down on the soft carpet of their foyer, figuring (as one of his medical sources had suggested) that this would make it easier for paramedics to perform CPR chest compressions if needed. A police officer was the first to arrive, and when my dad heard the knock he hollered at him to come in. When Mom heard the door open, she came downstairs in just a bra. The officer didn't seem to notice. But Dad did.

"Hey, love," he said quietly. "Go put a dress on." She ran back upstairs.

An EMS crew came next. And Mom reappeared, still undressed, this time carrying a shoe.

"This?" she asked my father, who was sitting amid the medical team attending him.

"No," Dad said. "Clothes."

She headed back up to their bedroom. No one made a move to help her. A paramedic scanned Dad's EKG reading and put an intravenous line in his arm. Mom came and went in different states of undress, flustered and confused. Dad lost track of her, an uncommon departure from his usual vigilance, though he did brief the group about her dementia. Somehow she made it to the front seat of the ambulance fully clothed as they sped away, siren wailing.

He spent that day and night in the hospital so doctors could observe and monitor him. He called their friend Sheelah to pick Mom up and take her to their house for a sleepover. After numerous tests—"too many," Dad said later when he called to let me know—doctors found no evidence of a heart attack. It had been purely stress- and anxiety-induced.

"You need more help," I told him. "This is not okay. This is a wake-up call, Dad."

"It's not a wake-up call. It's a pulled pectoral muscle," he grumbled. "I knew it wasn't a heart attack."

My frustration was growing. I wanted to give him the benefit of the doubt. I could only imagine what it was like to be in his shoes. I admired his instinct to care for my mother, to be a hero, to watch over her at all times. But he was losing perspective and common sense. I had held him up on a pedestal my whole life. He had always been my smart, strong, calm, centered father. Now, for one of the first times in my life, I realized that he was making foolish decisions and didn't know it.

I READ STUDIES ONLINE ABOUT the mental and physical risks of full-time caregiving. I learned that people like my father are vulnerable to multiple health problems: compromised immune systems, serious infections, depression, and even cognitive decline. He needed more help, and he still wouldn't admit it. I was starting to see that we were in danger of losing not only our mother but our father as well if we didn't act.

From the second I spotted them in baggage claim when they visited a couple months later, I could tell by my parents' faces that something was wrong. Other arriving New York passengers stared down at the conveyer belt, willing it to come to life and deliver their luggage. My mother was distracted, looking around for something she couldn't name.

Before even saying hello, Dad whispered, "Can you help your mom in the ladies' room?" He passed me a wrinkled plastic Holiday Inn laundry bag and nodded toward the restroom sign. Mom didn't say hello, either. She just giggled and shrugged at me as if to say, *Isn't this weird?*

I'd imagined that this trip to Nashville would give me and my brother a chance to learn more about her current state and to bear some of my father's caregiving burden. *He'll take naps and have time to write,* I'd hoped. *Maybe take a drive with Brad . . .*

But like many moments to come, none of what I expected happened. I glanced into the bag. Perhaps five hours before, when they'd left their house in New York, it had contained everything Mom needed for two and a half hours in the air. But now the supplies Dad packed had dwindled down to one pair of giant-looking tan underpants and one Ziploc baggie with a few sheets of rumpled tissue. It was as if he'd just pushed me off a cliff with a paper parachute. *Really?* I wanted to say.

"Let's go!" I said instead, as brightly as possible. "We'll be back in a second." I steered Mom by the elbow toward the ladies' room. We passed a few other women as I led her to the handicapped stall farthest from the door. She stood facing me. I handed her the skimpy bag.

"I'll wait right here," I said, backing out of the stall.

"What," she said. "What." She waited for me to understand something.

"You want me to come in?" She held out her hand to me, and I realized: *She doesn't know what to do.*

My dad had likely begun dealing with incontinence at home without telling us. It was up to me to take his place here, with no more warning than he'd had the first time. This abrupt initiation into the world of intimate, hands-on caregiving felt clumsy and awkward.

My mother had wet herself through her khakis, probably right after the plane landed. She unbuckled her belt but sat down on the toilet with her pants on.

"Oh, wait a minute," I said, as if I had just come up with an interesting idea. "Let's get these off first." I held her hands. She'd gained some weight, and it was difficult to stand her up because she didn't understand what I was trying to do. I pulled down her damp pants and underwear. She giggled. To my amazement, Mom was trying to make this moment easy for us by keeping it funny.

"Oof!" she said as she landed back down on the seat, halfway to a pratfall. I kept smiling as I dialed Dad on my phone. He didn't answer. I needed dry clothes from a suitcase. If I left her alone to get them, she wouldn't be able to lock the door after me. She could wander off into the terminal with her pants around her ankles. My mind raced.

Should I get her dressed and take her back outside wearing the wet clothes, or abandon her while I try to find Dad? I wouldn't leave my child here like this.

But she is an adult.

But in some ways, she's like a child.

And what if Dad hasn't picked up their bag yet?

Mom had stopped laughing. It was quiet in the bathroom. We were alone for the moment. I took my chances.

"I need to get you something else," I said. "I'll be right back."

"Okay!" she said, still managing a smile. I left her in the stall with the door open and broke into a jog toward the baggage claim, calling my father again. This time he answered.

"Dad!" I said. "Quick! I need her clothes!"

"Sure," he said. "I've got the bag—"

I hung up on him. *No time to talk,* I thought, panic start-ing to rise with each second my mom was alone in that stall. Moments later I reached him and he passed me some fresh clothes from her suitcase. I raced back to the restroom.

Someone was in another stall when I got there, and I didn't know if my mother had made friends with her from her toilet throne. But I was relieved to see Mom in the same place I'd left her, still smiling.

We didn't talk about what happened on the way to our house, or any other time. But the incident led my dad to learn that many airports and other public places have "family restrooms" to accommodate parents and children, as well as both genders at the same time. From then on, he would find them online before they left home so he'd know how to get to them quickly. And he would always pack a full change of clothes for Mom and plenty of cleanup supplies in their carry-on bags. Later he'd even figure out how to change her in the backseat of a rental car in a parking lot, as well as in the cramped lavatory of a plane while other pas-sengers wondered what the two of them were doing in there.

DURING THIS TRIP THEY STAYED in our guesthouse on the farm. They had their own bedroom and bathroom, which allowed them to come visit for longer periods, some-times weeks, while still giving us all some private space.

We gave Dad as much time off as we could. My brother picked up Mom for a walk or a ride in his truck. My friends Terri and Paula joined my mother and me for occasional lunches. Sandy and Jay's mother-in-law, Linda, took Mom shopping. Nana and Huck, who was three by then, spent time together often, in the playroom at our cabin, while I sat nearby supervising with Jasper in my arms.

She bought Huck a jack-in-the-box on one of our shopping trips. The two of them wound it up again and again, and shrieked when the clown sprang out of the box.

"Pop goes the weasel!" Mom still knew the lyrics.

"Again!" Huck yelled. And they did it over and over.

In another game, he would sit in her lap and tell her, "Nana, say 'Jasper.'"

"Ssss. Spasper!" she'd answer. She wasn't able to get his name out more clearly than that, and she and Huck would both crack up over their invention of a game born out of her disability.

One day Mom stopped laughing during the "Spasper" game and got quiet and sullen. She let us know she wanted to go home. We called Dad to pick her up and take her back to the guesthouse. She left our cabin coldly, with many words unsaid. My father called a few minutes later.

"Huck hurt your mom's feelings," he said. "She doesn't want to play that game anymore. I think it would help if you brought him over here to apologize." I felt as if I were hearing from the parent of another toddler that my son was a bully on the playground.

"What changed?" I asked. "She used to love it."

Dad admitted he had always been a little uneasy when his grandson made fun of Mom, even though she'd always been able to laugh at herself.

"I think she never really liked the game but she was playing along to make Huck happy," he said. Dad was treating her sadness as though it were rational. I swallowed my instinct to point out that Huck was three and that bringing her anger to his attention would only highlight her shortcomings for him. He was the only one in her world now who genuinely loved playing with her, who didn't see her as sick or odd, just fun and silly. Making him apologize would take away a measure of innocence and teach him what we hadn't had to yet: *Nana is different and needs to be treated delicately.*

I had to figure out a way to make sense of it for Huck.

"You're not in trouble," I told him. "But Nana has difficulty talking sometimes. And the game you play together hurts her feelings." He stared at me, uncomprehending. "She actually wishes that she could say Jasper's name, but she really can't. Do you understand?" He nodded, looking confused. "Do you think you could try to help her feel better?"

We practiced an apology together, and then found Mom, sitting in the guesthouse on the couch next to my father with her arms crossed. Her face was wet with tears. When she saw my son, she glared at him. He stopped and stared. He seemed to have forgotten the words we'd rehearsed. I nudged him.

"Sorry, Nana," he mumbled.

"Okay," she said quietly. He looked to me, and I nodded. *Yes, good. Keep going.* He approached her warily, hugged her, and then stepped back. In a matter of minutes, she'd changed from a loving and fun pal to a frightening, angry old lady. I ached for the pain and confusion both of them felt.

"We need to find new ways to have fun with Nana," I told him later that night. But even I didn't really know what that meant. Was there any more fun to be had? Where was my real mother? I was losing sight of her. But my firstborn somehow accepted this and took it to heart, determined to try.

Months after that, during another visit, Huck grabbed a picture book called *Snowmen at Christmas* off the shelf in his bedroom. He handed it to Mom, who was sitting on the floor.

"Nana, will you read this to me?" he asked. She looked to me in a panic, reluctant to admit to him that she couldn't anymore. *Help. I'm in over my head.*

But before I could say anything, Huck picked up on her discomfort.

"You can just make up a story from the pictures instead of reading," he told her.

"Oh! Okay!" she said. "Uh . . ." She hesitated again, holding the open book in her lap. Huck snuggled into the crook of her arm, patient, waiting. Then Nana plunged in, doing the only thing she could think of in that moment. She started tapping him on the top of his head and making train noises.

"Choo-choooo!" she said. *Tap. Tap. Thump.* The book fell off her lap and closed shut on the floor. "Ho!"

Huck caught my eye from beneath his grandmother's palm. *We need to find new ways to have fun with her.* I was astonished to see his eyes sparkling. He knew what to do.

"Good job," he said to her. She beamed.

AT HOME IN NEW YORK, various people took turns staying with Mom overnight so Dad could occasionally get some rest at a Catholic convent for twenty-four to forty-eight hours. In contrast to the chaos and mess at home, the convent rooms, with their cinder-block walls, were clean and small, and the self-imposed silence and peace appealed to him.

But the more other caregivers filled in for my father, the less happy they were to do it again. It was exhausting, hard work, and no one could understand how my dad had been handling so much by himself for so long. Ash hosted Mom in California for several weeklong stays. But my sister got so drained from these visits that she had to stay in bed for days afterward. My mother needed constant entertainment and wasn't content with being put in front of the television or being sent away for a nap. She had the attention span of a five-year-old but the pride of a matriarch. Though she enjoyed the overnights with friends, with her sister, with Ash, she raged at my father every time he told her he needed to leave again. She got mad at everyone at some point for one reason or another, but Dad got it the most. Often it infuriated her that he couldn't decipher her scrambled thoughts.

"What about that?" She would point at their television. It was turned off, the flat screen black.

"Do you want the TV on?" he would ask, reaching for the remote.

"No!" she'd yell.

"Something about a program?"

"No, it's *that*!" she'd say, still pointing at the screen. Dad likened her mind to a coatroom where all the coats lay in a messy pile on the floor. She was making less and less sense.

And she was having more and more accidents. Bruises, scrapes, and cuts on her arms and legs were starting to mark a trail of injuries. More than once she wound up in the emergency room, where Dad would have to speak for

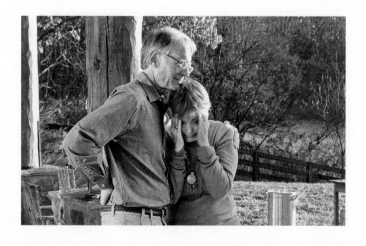

her. *She slipped on a wet bathroom floor. . . . She tripped on a crack in a sidewalk. . . . She bumped into a glass door. . . . She has primary progressive aphasia. Have you heard of it?*

MY MOTHER TOLD MY FATHER she couldn't take it anymore—she wanted to leave him. She badgered him and spewed insults at him for no clear reason, until occasionally he broke and raised his voice at her, a rare occurrence for him. She would be contrite for a day or so after, but Dad was depleted. By the end of 2010, the friends-and-family plan was fizzling out. Just trying to keep track of who was willing to step in to do what when was time-consuming.

We urged him to hire someone professional on a regular basis for many hours a week, whether Mom liked it or not. Dad said he wanted to but didn't know the most practical way of doing it, and felt as if he might be better off continuing to try to juggle his time and Mom's moods. In his kids' minds, his judgment was still way off.

It was time for a face-to-face intervention. We needed to take control of the situation. Jay, Ash, and I planned a trip home that winter. We gave my father a heads-up that we were coming to try to convince both of them to get more help, and he agreed to it, as long as we took the lead. Ash talked to an intervention specialist, and we came up with a plan. We would tell our mom that we were worried about Dad's health, and try to enlist her assistance in getting it for him. This would take the focus off our mother's limitations and put it onto our father. Still, all of us assumed we'd have to fight her on it.

Coincidentally, because of the way our schedules lined up, I would not be home for Huck's fourth birthday. I'd never missed his birthday before, and I felt awful about it. I knew he was only four and he probably wouldn't remember, but I also resented having to miss it. Then I hated myself for feeling resentment. I was torn by guilt over my responsibilities, both as a parent and as a daughter. There was no question that the talk in New York would have a greater impact if my brother and sister and I were all there in person as a unified team. It was where I had to be.

Still, I dreaded the visit. My siblings and I had never before fought to take charge of a Williams family crisis. It had always been Dad's role, or less frequently Mom's. I was very uncomfortable usurping his leadership, even though he'd admitted that he couldn't do everything by himself. The little girl inside me was also scared of my mother—of her unpredictable reactions, of her rage and despair, of the disease that was running our lives.

After Brad and I put the boys to bed the night before I left for the visit, my husband held me as I wept big gut-wrenching tears in bed. He had never seen me cry that hard.

"I'm so sorry," he said, again and again.

BUT THE TRIP ENDED UP going surprisingly well. Mom was overjoyed that we were all together, which then colored the tone of our confrontation. We had a group session with our father's therapist, Lynn Evansohn, who was also in on the plan. All three kids each explained how we were worried about him. By the end of the meeting, our mother had miraculously agreed to interview some in-home helpers that afternoon. Later, in our parents' living room, the five of us talked to two separate candidates available for part-time work who'd been sent from the senior living community nearby. Mom sat mostly silent as the rest of us asked questions.

JAY: "Have you been trained in cardiopulmonary resuscitation?"
ASH: "Do you like to cook?"
ME: "Do you have children?"

We weren't looking for specific answers so much as trying to get a feel for personalities. Afterward we convinced our mother that one of the women seemed sweet and fun. "She's a lot like Anna," we told her, knowing how much Mom adored her dear friend. She reluctantly agreed to give it a try. The next day, we stuck around while her new nurse's aide, Millie from Ghana, arrived for her first day on the job. She was everything we'd hoped for: outgoing and loving, with the many good qualities of Anna and Mom's other friends.

Largely because of Millie, we were able to get away alone with Dad to another caregivers conference at Northwestern that spring. He wanted to give it another try if we were there to do it with him. We still hoped for some new insight as to how to better handle PPA.

"Senior care" companies, offering free tote bags, buttons, and water bottles, lined the tables along the hall outside the auditorium where we sat inside, listening to lectures and young social workers telling us to take care of ourselves. We learned more by talking with other families, but over-all drew little relief from the gathering. I was struck by the looks of empathy I got from people whose loved ones had already died. Their eyes said, *There is no easy way through this. It sucks.* We asked a daughter who'd lost her father a year earlier when she knew it was the right time to put him in an assisted-living facility.

"You'll just know," she said. Her answer was infuriatingly vague. And I couldn't help envying her. She was already done with this hideous disease, and in a position to counsel others on how she survived.

THE NEXT FEW TIMES MY parents came to visit, we hired help in Nashville, too. But because Mom and Dad were there irregularly, the aides were different from visit to visit and even day to day. Few of them had much experience dealing with someone as challenging as my mother. They burned out quickly.

One day Dad left Mom at the guesthouse with a helper and came to visit me at our cabin. I opened a bottle of wine and put out some cheese on a plate. It was heavenly to celebrate a few simple minutes together with my father. We were almost giddy as he relaxed and allowed himself to be away from Mom for a little bit. We were watching the kids play in the yard when the phone rang. It was the aide, very upset. She asked my father to come back right away. When we got there, the woman was outside the house, pacing and crying.

"She hit me," she said.

It was a game-changer. We had been warned that Mom could become violent, but this was the first time she had ever struck anyone. We'd finally gotten my parents to accept help. Now that solution presented its own set of problems. Though we apologized and felt awful about what had happened, that person left. We never saw her again.

DAD AND JAY TOOK MOM out to dinner later at a Japanese fusion restaurant near the farm. My father ordered her a rainbow roll. The food came, and they started to eat.

Suddenly my mother yelped, stuck out her tongue, and stood up at the table.

She'd accidentally eaten a bean-sized chunk of wasabi, the searing Japanese mustard. As a few patrons around their table turned to look, Dad calmly held out a glass of water. Mom slapped it away, spilling it, and sat back down. She spit the wasabi out onto her plate with a puking sound.

A waiter appeared with a glass of milk. Jay held it up to her mouth.

"This will help," he said. It seemed to. She settled back down.

Without missing a beat, Dad carried on with the conversation. "What are the feelings about the election around here these days?"

Jay was dumbfounded. My father had developed a maddening ability to pretend nothing had happened after a crisis with Mom. It drove my brother crazy. It was a survival instinct, a desire to help protect my mother's pride to the end. *If we don't acknowledge it, it didn't happen.*

Because Mom's short-term memory was dimming all the time, she, too, went back to eating as though nothing had happened. Within seconds she put the very same chunk of hot mustard back into her mouth.

"Ahhhhh!" she shrieked again, louder this time. She pushed back her chair, got up, and started making her way around the table in a panic, howling as she walked. All eyes in the restaurant turned toward her. Dad coolly picked up the half-drunk glass of milk and followed after her.

"Try this," he said.

"Noooo!" she wailed, her face flushed.

Jay watched this scene with growing concern. He knew my dad's approach wasn't working.

So my brother did the only thing he could think of: He got behind my mother and grabbed her waist in a bear hug, the way he had learned as a firefighter to rescue people in emergencies. Carrying her with her feet a few inches off the floor as she shrieked, he took her to the exit, past shocked diners, speechless waiters, and astonished sushi chefs. Mom was hitting her head and crying.

"Thanks-for-coming-have-a-nice-night!" the hostess said, barely glancing up, as Jay shuffled our mother out the door.

My brother called me that night and recounted the story. We moaned with embarrassment and howled with laughter.

"No more restaurants," Jay said, and I agreed. From then on we would cook in or order takeout when Mom was around. Both of us were troubled yet again by how little an incident like this affected our father.

AFTER THAT VISIT, I WROTE an email to Dad, sharing my siblings' reactions to the visit and the current situation.

"This last trip to Nashville was the hardest yet," I said. I made a case for twenty-four-hour care. We were fortunate enough as a family to be able to afford that kind of help, at least in the short term. I thought that by hiring an additional person or two for around-the-clock care—someone well vetted who was used to caring for someone like Mom, who could maybe even travel to Tennessee with them—we might finally have a real break. But even in suggesting it, I wasn't sure that person existed. In the back of my mind, I was beginning to think my mother would be better off in a long-term facility. But along with that thought was the fear that she would be rejected, based on her growing aggression and complex care needs.

I was surprised when Dad wrote me back in agreement.

"She is increasingly crazy," he said.

And though I hadn't mentioned it to him directly, we were both hoping that in the face of her erratic and difficult behavior, the decision to move her out of their home would soon be made for us.

One day in the summer of 2011, Mom went missing.

There was a lot more missing in my life that record-hot season. I'd been raised to hope, to *believe*. I'd always trusted that good things or divine revelations could come from any crisis. Now Mom's losses were my losses, and that faith suddenly felt like a convenient cliché, a cruel joke. Gone was my quest to find the silver lining in our family's situation. I felt powerless, cynical, bitter. *How could I have been so naive?*

That was what I was thinking on the day Mom couldn't be found. It was the beginning of the time when everything got even worse.

Mom and Dad were in Tennessee for a few days, and Dad had driven her to our cabin. He watched her walk through the front door, assumed that she was fine, and drove away.

I was in the basement with my sister, who was also visiting, and we didn't know Mom had arrived. Ten or fifteen minutes after we'd been expecting her, I called my father.

"I dropped her off ten minutes ago," he said with alarm.

Ash and I searched the cabin. "Mom? Where are you?" She had disappeared.

Our voices echoed off the hardwood logs. We ran outside into the heavy summer heat and hollered, and again our cries seemed to mock us, ricocheting off the valley walls. There was no place else to look near my house. I got into the car and drove down the long, hilly driveway toward the guesthouse.

I rounded a curve and saw her, shoulders hunched, moving gingerly ahead of me. I caught up to her and realized that she'd taken off her sneakers, and she was clutching them to her chest. She was walking on the hot pavement in her socks. Her face was pink.

"You! Left me!" she spat at me when she saw me. I jumped out of the car and ushered her into the passenger seat to drive her home. But it was all I could do not to cry out what I had been feeling as never before: *No! You have left* me.

MY FATHER, A FORMERLY DEVOUT Episcopalian, said he had started to feel spiritually anemic. He really didn't know what he believed anymore. One day at the convent where he took his retreats, he saw a black-robed priest standing far ahead of him on a trail overlooking the Hudson. Dad turned away to avoid him. He didn't even want to say hello for fear the priest would want to talk. My father worried he might have to confess that he didn't have much faith left. That he was unable to take care of his wife. That although he had once made binding wedding vows before God and many witnesses, he was struggling in his soul with two words.

In sickness.

Mom's screams of "I hate you!" at my father echoed down their block in New York. Dad got calls from neighbors who'd seen her storm out of the house.

"She's on the move," they'd say.

"Thanks, I'm tracking her," he'd reply, grabbing his keys.

At night Mom got out of bed every couple of hours, usually pulling off the adult diaper Dad had put on her and relieving herself on the covers, the carpet, the door frame, the

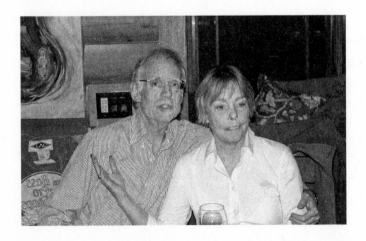

bathtub. Dad scrambled after her, groggy and numb, trying to clean up every bodily substance she left behind.

"Go away!" she yelled, followed by demonic-sounding yowling. Occasionally she threw things at him. Later she would be contrite, apologetic, though not fully knowing what she'd done wrong, like a child.

I resented my former mother, the woman I could barely remember now, who had left us with this mess. Why hadn't she set up a more specific caregiving plan when she knew enough to understand the disease was going to get worse? She should have made a list of examples—bathroom accidents and aggression would have been at the top—to clarify what she meant when she told my sister in 2005 that she didn't want Dad to take care of her. And she should have spelled out what she meant by "take care of." Dad thought he *was* getting help with caregiving, and more than that, he still felt bound to the promise he had made to her that he would never ask her to live outside their home, away from him. Now that promise was haunting him.

I seethed. I was mad at Dad, too. How could he let her walk all over him? How could he let this disease kill both of them? I turned forty, and for the first time in my life, I didn't hear from my parents at all on my birthday. I had a pit in my stomach. They'd abandoned me. And once again I hated myself for that selfish thought.

. . .

A COUPLE OF DAYS AFTER Thanksgiving that year, I got a message from Aunt Diana that my cousin Stephen was in a hospital in Raleigh with what doctors thought might be toxic shock syndrome. He was in critical condition.

"We need prayers," she said.

I offered up a quick one—to what felt like just myself.

I sent word to the family. Dad relayed the message to Mom, who wanted to leave for North Carolina immediately. She understood something was happening, but she didn't quite know what it was. By the next morning, she was furious with my father. She wanted to go somewhere, anywhere, and she couldn't. She sat by the door in her quilted red coat, a green wide-brimmed hat in her lap. She stared out a window, seething, patting her hat with one hand, waiting to go, like a boxer between rounds. Dad knew that at any moment she'd launch into her next round with him.

Feeling helpless, I tried to conjure up that eight-year-old pure-hearted girl who'd once implored a star to protect her from skidding toward a crash on an icy hill. I shivered. I got on my knees and asked for strength and healing and smart doctors. I didn't know if I'd been heard, but I did it anyway because Aunt Diana had asked me to.

Brad and I made two quick trips to North Carolina from Tennessee in the course of the ten days Stephen spent battling what turned out to be a severe strep infection. The second trip was to say goodbye.

His five-year-old son, Tyler, played in a small conference room down the hall with Beth's parents while the rest of us—

Bill, Diana, Beth, Brad, Jay, and I—held vigil at Stephen's bedside with his minister, Mike. We rubbed his arms and legs and talked to him for hours, though he was unresponsive. It felt interminable. I thought about my mother. How she should've been here, how she wanted to be. I was her second-team replacement. This wasn't supposed to be the order of things. We had thought we knew our enemy, the disease we were fighting as a family. Stephen's sickness blindsided us.

Finally his heart monitor slowed. The blips on the screen were farther and farther apart. And then they stopped. He was gone.

Shaking and weak, I walked down the hall toward the bathroom alone, my sneakers still tacky from dialysis machine fluid that had leaked out onto the floor of Stephen's room at one point in the last couple of hours. I pushed open gray double doors and turned left down another hall, leading me to an unexpected sign: *Chapel*.

I took a deep breath and opened the door.

It was a small room with about eight chairs in a couple of rows. In the corner was a large cross, and kneeling in front of it was a woman. She turned and looked at me, and a smile spread across her face as though she'd been expecting me.

"Hi!" she said. She had dark brown skin and sparkling eyes and wore scrubs.

"Hi," I said, new tears welling up. "Can I join you?"

"Yes!" she said. "Do you want me to pray with you?"

"Yes, please," I said, sitting on a chair slightly behind her. It felt weird to be suddenly so intimate with a stranger.

But her kindness and my desperation created the perfect opportunity.

"What happened?" she asked.

"My cousin just died."

"What's his name?"

"Stephen."

She grabbed both of my hands in hers and bowed her head.

"Lord, we are praying for Stephen right now," she said. I slid forward off the chair onto my knees alongside her.

"We thank you for his life, Lord. Please be with Stephen's family now, God. May they feel your love, and know the power of your Holy Spirit." As she spoke, I felt as if I'd walked into a little miracle. As if, for the first time in a long, long while, God was sending me a message through this woman, a kind of angel.

He was saying, *I am still here.*

After she finished her prayer, we hugged and I thanked her.

"Are you on a break?" I asked. The woman giggled.

"No," she said. "I just ran in here for a minute." When I left, I noticed her abandoned cart full of supplies waiting outside the door.

DAD AND MOM ARRIVED A few days later for the funeral. She was more manic than ever. If she saw someone crying, she wailed. If someone laughed, she cracked up in hysterics.

She radiated an urgency that matched her confusion. She didn't fully understand what had happened but seemed greatly impacted by the weight of everyone else's emotion. On the way back to the hotel after the service and a reception, Dad was driving down Interstate 40 at about sixty-five miles an hour when Mom suddenly wanted to get out of the car. She screamed at him, unbuckled her seat belt, and opened the door. My father grabbed her arm while keeping one hand on the wheel, and was able to swerve toward an exit. Her actions could have killed them both.

At the hotel, she peed on the lobby floor.

STEPHEN'S DEATH SHOCKED US AND reminded us that each one of us was vulnerable. But within this sobering truth, the angel in the chapel gave me a new resolve. I wanted to be a survivor, living in the spirit.

CHAPTER

13

Daily life didn't leave much room for divine spirit. Without realizing it, I'd turned my mom into two different people: Old Mom and New Mom. New Mom was an unpredictable wild animal. One night she attacked my father at the top of a flight of stairs, screaming, "Get out! Shit! I hate you!" and pushed him hard in the chest, startling and scaring him.

New Mom needed to be treated with care and caution.

But held captive inside was her doppelgänger, Old Mom.

"You think I'm terrible," Old Mom said the morning after that tantrum, when Dad told her she'd crossed the line. She was quietly weeping, and he noted that she'd spoken a rare complete sentence.

"No, I don't," he said, and he meant it. He was talking to my real mother.

Occasionally she broke out and showed herself—in a

burst of genuine laughter or a funny expression I'd seen my whole life, one that I knew meant *Isn't this ridiculous?* I'd

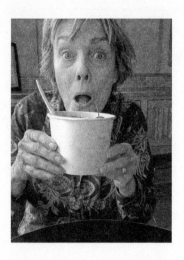

recognize her in her delight at eating a scoop of vanilla ice cream, or in her heavy sigh at seeing the ocean. She was the one who had once covered a wreath in bright white lights and hung it in the window of my darkened bedroom when I felt as if I were going to die at sixteen from mono. The one who had once gotten so engaged on the sidelines of my high school soccer game, jumping in the air and cheering so loudly we couldn't hear the ref. The one who made that soulful spaghetti and meat sauce I loved, and reassured me after a hard day by saying, "It'll make a great story one day."

A good story wouldn't ever fix her. Old Mom tormented me, wounded me with her silence, and sometimes left me sobbing in bed for hours. She was like a ghost who was fading fast. The harder I tried to grasp her, the more it felt as if she'd deserted me. New Mom was a cruel counterfeit, reminding me that the other one wasn't gone, wasn't at peace, but was trapped. While I treasured rare glimpses of who she used to be, I also felt haunted. I kept wanting to say out loud, *If you could see yourself now, Mom, you'd want to die.*

EARLY IN 2012, WE WERE all dealing with different degrees of guilt about what we could and couldn't do anymore for her. My dad was sharply focused on the secret he was keeping from her: He'd finally started considering options for long-term care.

The guilt I carried was about urging him in that direction. I felt like I didn't have an ounce of his patience. The truth I hated to admit was that I couldn't stand to be around my mother anymore.

I'd been talking more often with my therapist, Karen, in California. I'd started seeing her off and on when I'd moved to Los Angeles right after college, and she'd been instrumental in teaching me how to become a healthy grown-up.

Karen is a joyfully spiritual person who loves to celebrate everyday life with glitter—in her short spiky hair, on her face, on her nails. She smells of sweet perfume and sports a small sparkling nose ring. She laughs easily and often, and at the same time points unapologetically to the hard lessons. For years she's kept a little pillow on her couch that reads, *If it's not one thing, it's your mother.*

Karen had watched and helped guide my evolving relationship with Mom. A long time ago, she'd shed light on the ways my mother attached her needs to mine, so that I sometimes felt as if I had to take care of her, and had to fight to make my own choices.

Everybody I've ever met has had some sort of issue with one or both of their parents. It's what keeps therapists employed. And I have no doubt that one day Huck and Jasper will complain about the mistakes I've made. But Karen and I didn't harp too much on the past. We talked a lot about moving forward.

"Turn anger into compassion, and fear into faith," she told me more than fifteen years ago. I scribbled it down on a yellow Post-it note and stuck it into my Filofax. For a long time, it was my mantra.

These days we were delving deeper into forgiveness, of New Mom for her behavior and of myself for my resentment. Whatever issues I still had with my mother were mine alone to handle. I'd hoped for an epiphany—that Mom would one day say, "You know, I really overreacted to your engagement to Brad" or "I regret letting fear overcome me when I got diagnosed" or even "Gee, I may have struggled with anger and a bit of depression when you were little." But I had to accept I'd never hear her say those words.

We talked about long-term care. I told Karen I thought it was fair to assume that Old Mom, at her best, would be screaming at us to save my father's life. Karen's answer surprised me. Conjecture about what my mother would have said under different circumstances was irrelevant.

"We have to look at what *is*," she said. Bottom line: Dad couldn't see it, but the current situation had to change. With Karen's prompting and encouragement, my siblings and I and our spouses scheduled another telephone intervention with my father.

"Be clear about your agenda and intentions for the call," Karen said. "Give everyone a chance to speak." We would outline for my dad our concerns, using specific examples. We would present possible solutions. We would suggest a follow-up plan. We set up a date for our phone meeting with my father in early March. He arranged for someone to be with my mom.

With everyone in three states linked on a conference call, Brad told my dad about an incident when my parents had visited us in our house north of Los Angeles. We were getting ready to go for a drive, and I'd handed my two-year-old off to my father when he asked how he could help.

"Can you please put Jasper in his car seat?" I said, and walked back into the house.

But Dad got distracted when he saw my mom wandering around in our front yard, crying. He sensed that she was on the verge of a meltdown. He put Jasper down in the driveway, next to the road where cars raced by, and walked away. When Brad came out a minute later, he was horrified to find our son alone so close to the street.

My father didn't have much memory of this incident when we recalled it, and he felt awful. We told him about another low point during that visit, when Huck and I had found my mother banging on the glass windows in the house, frantic to get out. She didn't know how to use the front door right next to her.

She'd recently been prescribed a little pink pill called Seroquel, which was normally used as an antipsychotic. The drug was a lifesaver, although Dad was a slave to the timing of the dosage. I told my father that I'd seen in California what she was like when he was a little late in administering it: For the first time, I'd witnessed her babbling in anguish, totally unaware that she wasn't making any sense.

We laid out once again how concerned we were for Dad's health and safety. We told him again that he seemed vacant, depressed, lost.

"We really miss you," we said. "Even when we're with you."

Jay and I offered to look into long-term care in Tennessee, where the cost of living was lower than New York's and my parents could be closer to their grandkids and us.

"It's time to rip off the Band-Aid," Jay said, meaning it was going to hurt all of us to move her somewhere else, but it had to happen. We were relieved at the end of the call when Dad finally said, "I agree."

Jay and I started looking at "memory care"—dementia—facilities in Tennessee. I called a friend in the medical profession in town for a suggestion. My mother-in-law put me in touch with a friend of hers whose older parent had been put into assisted living in the area. My brother and I came up with a short list between the two of us.

The first place we visited reminded me of my grandmother's nursing home from almost thirty years before. It smelled like overcooked lima beans and diapers. There were no windows in the main sitting area, where residents dozed in front of a *Jeopardy!* rerun on a flat-screen TV. Two women, with paper bibs tucked into their shirts, sat at a small square dining table. They stared ahead, one with a half-empty cup of coffee in front of her and the other with a bowl of untouched applesauce. Neither spoke. All of the residents looked older than my mother by about ten years. We left feeling depressed.

Another community was a little more cheerful. As we walked into the sunny living area—there were plenty of windows here—an upbeat female resident was playing the piano. She said hello as we passed by. Although the men and (mostly) women living in this place also seemed older than my mom, many appeared generally happy, or at least placid.

We checked out a room where a handful of residents were assembled for a current events symposium. Newspapers lay strewn on the tables and on a couple of laps. A younger worker at the front of the room was leading a discussion by reading the paper aloud. Some listened patiently, others slept. One man barked passionate opinions.

"That's mutiny," he said. "My head's wrapped around that one. That's the one."

"You think so?" said the discussion leader, nodding as though he'd made a really good point.

We told our tour guide a little about Mom.

"So she can't speak?" the woman said.

"Not much, no."

"Is she able to show where she has pain?" she said.

We hesitated. "Well, not necessarily."

Turned out that was a problem. She couldn't be accepted there unless she was able to communicate.

In New York, Dad also encountered a glitch in his search for a place. The assisted-living residence that supplied Millie and other home health aides for my parents told him that if my mother were admitted, she'd have to spend a couple of weeks in a psychiatric ward first to get her meds worked out—meaning she'd have to be sedated enough to prevent attacks on other residents or staff. My dad couldn't bear the idea of sending her from home to a hospital bed.

Other places he looked at were similar to the ones Jay and I toured. Dad got very sad in one of them, watching an exercise class led by two adults for more than a dozen quiet residents, most of them older than Mom and all of them seated.

One of the residents introduced herself to my father.

"Hi, I'm Spunky," she said. "All the people here are boring. And stupid."

Finally, though, after seeing three communities close to home, Dad visited a place about fifteen minutes from Rye that had opened recently and could pass for a good hotel. Because it was new, it still had a vacancy. A friendly woman greeted visitors at the reception desk and kept watch over the two-story-high hall. Its centerpiece, at the foot of a dramatic staircase to an upper floor, was a gleaming grand piano. A rainbow-colored jukebox was playing "Boogie Woogie Bugle Boy of Company B," the Andrews Sisters hit from 1941, the year Dad was born. Patients like Mom didn't live on this floor, though. They were on the locked-down fifth level, which offered the most intensive care.

My father was invited into a small conference room. He sipped decaf coffee at a table with Sarah, the director of family services, as well as the executive director, Courtney. He knew by now that the first visit to any such community involved a sales pitch, and staff members would be on their best behavior. So it was important to see beneath the glitz. But these women seemed remarkably down-to-earth.

"Tell us about Linda," Sarah said.

"We've been married forty-five years," my father said. "Until recently, she's been my close partner in everything."

They wanted to know about him. "How do you feel?"

He was tired, he said. "My grandson told me I look old."

"What will you do after she enters long-term care?"

"I want to go away. Be alone."

He wondered, *What do they think of me?* He scanned their faces. Sarah's eyes were filled with tears. Her father had died of dementia. The questioning continued. For one of the only times since Mom's diagnosis, my dad cried.

They brainstormed with him about how he could break the news to his wife that she'd be leaving home.

"There is no formula," one of them said. "No easy way." Often families chose to stretch the truth about what was happening, opting instead for what they termed "fiblets," little white lies to help residents ease into the truth. *You're going to stay at this nice hotel for a week.* Or *Just try it to see if you like it.* Often this seemed the kinder way to go.

"We'll help you and Linda through this," they said. Furthermore, they'd be able to take her without an extended hospital stay first. Their advanced license allowed them to offer many of the services that nursing homes could. Mom would never have to move.

After two more visits, my father was sure he'd found the right place, but he knew he couldn't pay for it on his own. Brad and I offered to offset the cost of care, and that clinched it. He and I chuckled to ourselves over what Mom would've said all those years ago during our tense engagement if we'd told her that, on top of everything else, my future husband was going to be the one to make it possible to send her away one day. But my heart went out to all the many people in our situation who didn't have the means to even consider a choice like ours.

IT WAS SETTLED. DAD WOULDN'T be moving to Tennessee. Jay and I would miss having them close to us, but we realized that our father would probably adjust better if he stayed within his existing community. Mom was scheduled for the move less than two weeks later, in mid-April.

Aunt Diana flew in a couple of days beforehand, although Mom didn't yet know why. Ashley came home as well but hid at Sheelah's house, the site of my parents' retirement party years earlier. We didn't want my mother to realize what was happening until right before moving day. My father asked my brother and me not to be there, because he thought it would be harder on my mom if all of us showed up only to deliver her to a new place and leave her there alone.

I didn't fight him on this decision. I was filled with a mixture of guilt and relief. Guilt, because of course I wouldn't physically be there for one of the most difficult challenges we had ever faced as a family. And relief, because I wouldn't have to feel firsthand the pain of committing what felt like a great betrayal. I didn't realize how hard it would be to experience it secondhand, from so far away, as a powerless witness.

Ash and Diana surreptitiously filled a suitcase with Mom's clothes, shoes, and toiletries. They packed framed pictures of family and friends, and Mom's parachute book. They went to Kohl's and bought my mother some stylish new pants and a ten-dollar necklace they thought she'd like. They got her a bath mat and a colorful shower curtain. They bought her some dark chocolate.

While Dad took care of Mom at the house, they drove together to her new home and laid everything out in Mom's soon-to-be new bedroom with a large window, easy chair, and private bathroom. My sister and aunt decorated the walls with family photos and made up my mother's single bed with a rose-covered comforter—the one she and I had

picked out together for my grown-up bed when I was a teen-
ager. I remember how much we'd loved the floral print with
red and purple blooms and tiny dark green leaves, one of
the few things we'd agreed on when I was at that know-it-
all age. After we chose it, my mother surprised me with a
pretty pink teddy bear to finish off the look. That stuffed
animal rode on top of the rest of Mom's things. Ash laid it
on the comforter.

They hung pants and shirts in the closet, and the shower
curtain in the bathroom. They stocked the drawers of the
dresser with underwear and socks, and put the chocolate
on her pillow. *Just like a luxury hotel.*

The next day, while my father drove Diana to the airport, Ashley threw an impromptu dance party for Mom
and Sheelah in the foyer of my parents' house. They blew
out Dad's speakers playing Mumford and Sons. They tossed
lightweight scarves up into the air and watched them
float down like magic. Mom laughed with delight. Her joy
punched my sister in the gut. Were they making a huge
mistake? In many ways Mom was like an innocent child,
and what they were about to do—move her against her will—
could destroy her.

When Dad got home from the airport, he went to the
kitchen and got a simple anesthetic: a chocolate chip cookie.

"Scout, let's talk," he said, leading my mom to the couch
in the TV room and handing her the treat.

*And they had chocolate chip cookies and hot chocolate,
and that was the end.*

As she ate, he said, "You're getting stronger, and you've been getting better lately." A fiblet.

Ashley sat in the downstairs guest room, where she could best hear the conversation without being seen. She left the door ajar and texted me. In California, I sat on the floor of my bedroom, clutching my cell phone and shaking. I could hear my boys playing outside the door, unaware of what was happening to Nana in New York.

He's telling her, Ash wrote. *Oh, God.*

"I love you," Dad said. "And I want to get better care for you. I've found a place. It's like a luxury hotel—"

"No no no," my mother said, dropping the cookie and standing up.

"*Please* sit down," Dad said.

My mother said, "I love you" and "Don't." And then she left the room.

I didn't hear from my sister for a while after that. She went after Mom. It took a long time to settle her down, but eventually she slumped onto the floor at the bottom of their staircase. My sister huddled with her there.

"Give it a try," Ashley whispered.

"What happened?" my mom asked, weeping.

"Seven years ago you were diagnosed with a sickness called primary progressive aphasia...." She went on explaining the story to my mother again, as if for the first time.

·   ·   ·

LATER THAT DAY, ASHLEY CALLED me, crying. At first, it was hard for me to understand what she was saying through sobs. Then she said it clearly.

"She bit him," she said. "Dad was trying to give Mom her Seroquel and she bit him! Oh God oh God." She was pacing on the sidewalk outside their house. "I don't know what to do."

She began retching.

Lord, save us from this pain. I wept as I listened to her heaving two, three times. My little sister. My charge. The one I'd always told my secrets to and wanted fiercely to protect. Now there was nothing I could do but bear witness.

"I'm so sorry," I said. "I'm so, so sorry."

"I just threw up on the sidewalk," Ash said when she was done, as if I needed an explanation, and we both laughed for a moment about the absurdity of it all.

DAD SPENT MOST OF THE night in the upstairs guest room. Ashley set up a blanket and pillow on the floor of my parents' bedroom so she could help my mother when she needed it. When Dad realized that it might be the last time he'd ever sleep in the same bed with his wife, he got up, crossed through a hall to their room, and crawled in next to her. In the predawn hours, he held her, comforting her, and then added a blanket against the early morning chill.

14

D ad was familiar with the route to my mother's new home. But on the morning when he took her there for the first and last time, he drove cautiously, afraid that he might get lost. Next to him in the passenger seat, Sheelah chatted with Ashley, who sat behind her, barely aware of what she was saying. My sister kept her eyes on Mom, ensuring that she wouldn't unfasten her seat belt and once again try to get out of a moving car.

My mother began crying softly. Sheelah unwound a light white scarf from her neck and handed it to Ash to wipe Mom's tears.

"Scared," Mom said.

"That makes sense," Ashley said. "I'm scared, too."

They parked in the underground garage and met Sarah at the elevator. She welcomed my parents without a trace of institutional condescension. Mom was quiet, somber, weepy.

The fifth floor looked dreary. A few people slept sitting up in the living room. Sarah pointed to a petite short-haired woman in a wheelchair who was muttering to herself.

"Doctor, Ph.D.," she said. "She was teaching until recently."

"Oh," my mother said, shaking her head. She tried to negotiate her escape. The place was nice, she said, speaking in sentence fragments to convey the compliment. In a few polite but garbled words, she communicated that it was not quite right for her but she appreciated their efforts. She actually said, "Thank you."

My sister's doubt crept back. *Maybe this is a mistake. Mom is more lucid than she's been for months. She doesn't belong here.* The rooms seemed sterile compared with what Ashley had seen just a day before.

A man known on the floor as "The Diplomat" was wide-awake. Ashley liked him.

"There are two men standing behind you," he'd told her when she had met him for the first time a few days earlier. She'd turned around to look.

"I can't see them," she said.

"I can," he said. "That's because I have dementia." He was smart, and seemed to have a thirst for drama and adventure. Just like my mother.

With Mom by her side now, Ashley seized the opportunity.

"Hi," she said to the man. "This is Linda."

"Pull up a chair," he said, barely glancing at her. He was in his "office," which consisted of a desk near the entrance with an old but functioning typewriter. The *New York Times* was spread out in front of him. My mother sat down next to him.

My sister tried to engage him.

"What have you been up to?" she asked.

It didn't work. The Diplomat was busy and quiet. My sister tried again, but he wasn't in the mood, and neither was Mom. So they got up and headed down a hall to our mother's room, accompanied by a woman named Lisa, who was in charge of the floor.

Mom barely glanced at the decorations and homey touches my sister and aunt had chosen with care for her private space. She turned and walked out the door in search of Dad and Sheelah. Lisa started to follow. Ashley stopped her.

"What do we do?" she whispered. The question about how to break away on moving day had haunted her and Dad for weeks.

"You have to leave," Lisa said. "And it's gonna suck." *Time to rip off the Band-Aid.* By then, my sister had her emotions in check. Lisa made it clear that delaying the departure was increasing the pain. Driven by adrenaline, Ash left the bedroom, passed by our mother without saying a word, and strode the length of the hallway to an alcove at the exit. Lisa had given her the keypad code, 0911. The next step was the hardest.

"Hey, Dad," Ash called to my father. He didn't hear her. "Dad, can you come here?" She did the same with Sheelah. Sarah and Lisa distracted Mom, who hadn't noticed that everyone who'd brought her there had gone away. No one said goodbye.

Ashley's heart was pounding. She tapped 0911 quickly. As the door opened and they slipped out, they thought they heard my mother on the other side, running toward them. But they didn't look to find out. The door shut and its lock clicked. The elevator opened almost immediately. It was over.

Ashley broke down in tears as they descended. Sheelah tried to comfort her. Dad was silent.

My family had always made a big deal out of hello and goodbye, especially when we weren't going to see each other for a while. As he left the building, my father began the latest of many arguments with himself. *There must have been better and kinder ways to have left,* he thought. *But what good would any last hug or "I wish you well" or "I'm sorry" have done?*

When he got back home, drained, guilty, relieved, he went upstairs to their king-sized bed. He picked up his pillow from the right side and moved it to the center.

· · ·

AFTER THEY LEFT, MOM HAD in fact run after her friend, daughter, and husband, and just missed catching them at the exit.

"I think they went that way," Lisa told her, pointing my mother away from the door. Mom became hysterical. Various people tried to soothe her but failed. Her arrival was one of the most challenging ever at the facility, then and since.

Finally Sarah stood in front of her and said, "Linda, I *know* you can do this."

My mom stopped crying briefly and looked at her.

"Would *you*?" my mother asked. *Would you adjust to this abandonment? Would you force yourself to calm down in this godawful situation?*

Sarah thought for a moment.

"I am a wife, a mother, and a daughter, like you," she said. "And yes. Yes, I would."

My mother sighed deeply. Her panic subsided temporarily. She had a friend, someone who was listening, who took her seriously, who understood.

It was not the end of the trauma. Over the next few days Mom rattled doors and tied scarves around doorknobs, perhaps in the hope that they held the power to turn into keys and set her free. She lashed out at nurses and other residents. She wailed and was heavily medicated.

But, remarkably, within a few more days, she also began to laugh, and dance, and sing, and make connections. Mom had always loved people, and her floor was bustling with them. Besides the residents, there were warm caregivers—

certified nurse assistants with advanced training compared with most of the home health aides we'd hired. She was no longer trapped alone in her house with my father, who was exhausted and numb.

MY DAD BROKE HIS PLEDGE to himself about staying away for extended R&R and returned for a visit on the weekend after moving day. He was worried Mom would be mad at him, but instead was startled by how happy she was to see him. She was more herself than she'd been for months, holding hands with him and hugging, humming with pleasure when he scratched her back, laughing at his stories about friends and family.

But after his visit and one other from Anna, my mother relapsed into depression and panic, swinging between breathless, manic highs and angry, agitated lows. Once again the party was over and she hadn't gone home. So Lisa called for a two-week moratorium on visits.

Sarah kept us up to date. We clung to her stories and brief iPhone videos.

In one short clip she sent, Mom was sitting on the edge of a chair in the living room, clapping her hands and bouncing her feet while she listened to a sweet activities director named Edward sing and play the guitar. She looked cute with jean shorts and sparkling long earrings that swung as she moved. One of the residents, an older man, eyed her with interest from his wheelchair. She was blissful, and absentmindedly flicking the side of her nose with her fingers the way she always had. She looked up at Sarah, reaching out her hand, as if to say, *Put the phone down! Come listen! It's great!*

They didn't take videos of the harder times, though there were many more of those.

I came in early May, three weeks after the move. Lisa had reluctantly agreed we could give another visit a try, *if* Mom was having a good day. My mother could be combative, she told us, though her doctor was trying some new medications to stabilize her moods without making her too sleepy. We would have to see when I got there. I felt nauseated and light-headed as my father drove me to the home. I didn't want to make things harder for my mom, but I was dying to see her in person, to make sure she was okay, to tell her I loved her. I knew that at the last minute Lisa and Sarah might recommend that I just tour the facility and forgo a visit. If that were the case, I hoped maybe they would at least let me see her from afar.

But when we arrived, they said I could do it. Mom had been cheerful and seemed stable, and it was worth trying. We decided that Dad would remain in the lobby so my mother wouldn't see him, and I would proceed cautiously. If all went well initially and she still seemed happy, Mom and I would come down and have lunch together in the main dining room. Dad would hide behind his newspaper so she wouldn't see him as we passed.

I prayed I wouldn't make things worse for her. My mind

raced with questions. Would she be mad at me? Would she recognize me? Would it be hard to leave?

The staff would be crucial in getting me out the door when I was ready to go. Distraction was paramount. I took a deep breath to calm my nerves as Sarah punched the code into the keypad to let us in. The door unlocked with a click, and we entered Mom's world.

The floor reminded me of the facility that Jay and I had liked in Tennessee. It was clean, bright, and calm—homier than I had imagined from Ashley's description. Straight ahead in the dining area, people sat at tables finishing up lunch. Around the corner in the living room, there was a yoga class in progress. I scanned the space quickly but couldn't see Mom at first.

And then suddenly there she was, walking a little unsteadily in my direction. Her hair looked clean, parted on the side in a style I'd never seen before on her, as though someone who didn't know what she used to look like had taken great care in combing it. She was wearing a grayish-blue sweater and some pretty blue-and-white earrings to match. She didn't notice me.

"Hi, Mom," I said gently. She looked over, surprised.

"Kim!" she said, using my name for the first time in about a year. And then she started screaming.

"Ohhhh!" she cried, reaching for me. She grasped Sarah by my side. *This is my daughter,* she seemed to be saying. She was laughing, crying.

"I know! Kim's here!" Sarah said, sharing the enthusiasm.

"Ohhhh!" Mom yelled again, at full volume. She was making quite a scene, but my self-consciousness passed almost instantly. I realized anything goes in a place like this. It's full of people who are confused, manic, loud. It sank in: *This is the perfect place for my mother.*

She collapsed into me, sobbing.

"Hi," I said again, countering her exuberance with a deliberate calm. *Time to redirect.* I pulled away. "Hey, will you show me around?"

It worked. She clung to me, accidentally digging her pink nails into my forearm. A few days earlier, Sarah had sent us a picture of her daughter, who'd volunteered to give Mom a manicure. Some of the polish was messed up, most likely because Mom was unable to understand "hold still."

We walked toward the living room. Edward, the activities director from the video, greeted us.

"Hello, Linda!" he said. Mom had bonded with him, perhaps attracted to his British accent, much like her father's. And she loved hearing him play his guitar.

The yoga session was ending. He was about to begin. We found a spot on the couch. Edward strummed and started singing "What a Wonderful World." Mom was familiar with Louis Armstrong's raspy original rendition.

She listened thoughtfully to him, as though she were attending an opera, and then she began crying again silently. I pulled out my phone to take a video of her, and she looked over at me. She reached her hand toward the side of my face.

"You like this song?" I asked her.

"Yes," she said, tearing up. Then she noticed what I was doing.

"It's my phone," I explained, recording.

"So what?" she quipped. Though it didn't make sense, her tone told me she meant for it to be funny. I giggled.

Next up, Edward broke into "My Bonnie Lies over the Ocean," the old song my parents used to sing to us when we were kids. Mom loved this one, too.

"Bring back," he sang, "bring back, bring back my Bonnie to me, to me ..." I joined in. Behind us, a beautiful woman known on the floor as "Gertie the Birdy" for her pretty voice and elegance, sat up straight, remembering all the words and almost perfectly keeping up with the tempo. Edward strummed the final chord, and Mom took a deep breath and sighed happily.

"How about this one? I know you love this one, Linda," he said.

"Oh," she joked with him. "Pooh!" Meaning, I think, *What song* don't *I like?* Or perhaps *Are you flirting with me?*

He launched into "I Can See Clearly Now," the popular Johnny Nash song. "All of the bad feelings have disappeared..."

"Come on, Mom, let's dance," I said. I pulled her up with both hands.

"Wooo!" she cheered, shaking her hips. Then she was suddenly affectionate, pulling me into a hug and cradling her head into my neck.

"Shut up!" a disgruntled man behind us yelled. Mom shrugged at me as if to say, *He does that.* I shrugged back, smiling.

I took her to lunch downstairs in the dining room, walking right past Dad, who was buried behind his *New York Times*. We had some salad and soup, but neither of us ate much. I gathered up my courage to ask a burning question, afraid of what the answer might be or what it could trigger.

"So, Mom," I said as casually as I could, "you like it here?"

She answered without hesitating.

"I love it!" she said.

Miraculously, in that moment it seemed as if she meant it. *Was it as easy as that?* I needed to believe so.

noticed I'd started talking about my mother in the past tense.

"My mom loved lobster," I told someone over dinner at a seafood restaurant. "No, she didn't die," I clarified. Old Mom just wasn't there anymore.

My dad disagreed that she wasn't present. He told my mother's psychiatrist, Dr. B., what he guessed was on her mind: *I want to go home* or *My family has abandoned me* or even *I love it here*.

The doctor didn't think so. "Nothing like normal thinking is going on," he said. "She's all instinct."

Dad argued that he still saw flashes of her personality.

"Could be," Dr. B. said. "But they're probably coming from some lower part of her brain." Old memories, even old strategies that made people laugh–the equivalent of tricks or involuntary reactions.

I took what the doctor said to heart, because I saw it. Though the adjustment overall had been easier than we'd thought it would be, during her first spring there she scratched and knocked down a woman who was one of the few residents who also had primary progressive aphasia. My mother attacked the staff, too, more than once. Dr. B. scrambled to assemble a new mix of medications strong enough to blunt her aggression but gentle enough to allow her to stay awake and as active as possible. The heavier meds put her at great risk for falls and made her head droop forward like a dying flower. The loss of brain function was also weakening her muscle control.

The possibility that she might still have normal thoughts and fears that were hidden from us, that she might be feeling the pain and horror of her experience or understand what was happening to her, was unbearable. I preferred accepting the loss and trying to move forward. But to do that I needed to mourn, and I was having trouble figuring out how while she was still alive. I was in a holding pattern of confused grief.

The doctor guessed that, based on averages, she had two years to live, though no one could know for sure. *Two more years.* It felt like an eternity.

Visits to see her every couple of months or so were hard for me. I couldn't tell if she recognized me anymore or not. She'd not said my name since that first visit. I was relieved that she was largely someone else's responsibility now. But I still hated seeing her the way she was. From my perspective, the fifth floor was full of lost souls—angry and sad people trapped together with no hope of escaping except through death. It was bleak.

Yet I had to do it. She was—*is*, I had to remind myself—my mom, even if she didn't seem anything like it.

I brought Huck with me during Labor Day weekend, fearing that he might be devastated by the visit. That it would be heartbreaking for him to see his grandmother in the state she'd be in, that he wouldn't know what to make of the other residents. But he was unfazed when I tried to warn him. He was just excited to see her. He picked out his outfit by himself: an orange long-sleeved plaid shirt that buttoned down the front and a peach-and-blue striped clip-on tie.

"I want to look fancy for Nana," he said. He spiked up his hair in front with gel.

My dad had moved quite a bit of my mother's things out of the house in the months she'd been gone. Each time I came home, there was less of her there, but still I searched. I hoped to find something I hadn't seen before. A memory I hadn't revisited. A sign that she was still around. This time I looked under the bed. Had she left something there? No.

But the little round M. A. Hadley dish was still on the table in the guest room, where she'd put it years before. *A very Happy Easter to you* circled the edge in blue brush-strokes, surrounding a bunny with pink ears and mouth. It wasn't Easter, but the pottery had been on that table year-round for at least six years, quirky and warm, comforting and familiar. Mom had loved it and wanted guests to see it. *There she is,* I thought.

Her green canvas hat still hung on a hook by the back door. She used to wear it to protect her face outside. Dad hadn't needed to take it to her because she was rarely in the sun anymore.

I looked for a sign of her in the upstairs closet. It was still full of her things. Her faded Lanz of Salzburg nightgown, with the pattern of tiny red hearts and blue flowers, dangled down on the inside of the door. Had she hung it there? It still smelled like her. I took it off the hook and put it in my suitcase to hang in my own closet at home (where it still is now).

A yellow Post-it note she had left for my dad years before, when she could write, speak, and think, was still taped to the wall at the bottom of the stairs. I'd noticed it every time I was there.

I love you, it said in Mom's bold hand, with a smiley face.

Dad told me he explored the house, too, and clung to odd mementos. On the back of a shelf in the pantry, he stored one of the last grocery items she'd bought. It was mug cake mix in a small box. Stir water into it. Pour it into two coffee cups and microwave for one minute and twenty seconds. The box promised a pair of miniature chocolate cakes with glistening crusts. Mom must have figured that it would be easy for her to make the his-and-hers dessert she'd found for them. The mix had expired a year before, but Dad couldn't bring himself to throw it away.

MY FATHER DROVE HUCK AND me to her place.

My son smoothed his tie as we walked into the common area. Mom was sitting in a chair in front of the fireplace. Her head was down, so she didn't notice when we arrived. I knelt and looked up at her face.

"Hi, Mom," I said. "I brought Huck."

"Ooohhh!" she said, lifting her head as much as she could. She seemed delighted. Huck put his arms around her.

"Hi!" she said.

"Hi, Nana," he said, smiling. Someone on the other side of the room wailed. I winked at Huck. *People act differently in these places,* I'd told him earlier. *It's okay.* He smiled at me and turned back to my mom.

"Can we see your room?" he asked.

Her body language signaled an invitation. We walked with her down the hall and through her door. Huck loved the bed, which moved with the touch of a button. We helped her stretch out on top, and they laughed together as Huck made it go up and down, up and down.

When we said goodbye, she started to get sad, but Edward appeared with a song to distract her. Huck seemed content as we drove home. I was surprised and relieved that it hadn't been as traumatic for him as it usually was for me.

We came back a couple of months later with Jasper and Brad, and gained an extra family member. Tutti, another resident, usually seemed to think she was part of the kitchen staff. She was genuinely helpful, picking up plates and wiping off tables. As soon as she saw our three-year-old, she fell in love with him.

"Aren't you a cute little thing," she said to Jasper, reaching out and rubbing his cheek. He was polite. Tutti started following us around, "helping" us keep an eye on him.

"Be careful with that, honey," she said when Jasper picked up a rubber ball. "Come here. Come over here." His tolerance was beginning to fray. We retreated to Mom's room, but Tutti joined us.

When I was growing up, Mom was jealous of our time together. She didn't appreciate it when friends dropped by uninvited. But now she seemed blasé about letting Tutti sit on her bed next to her grandchildren during this precious visit. *What the hell?* We all rolled with it . . . until the end of our visit. We said our goodbyes, and Dad punched in the code to exit. Suddenly Tutti lunged at Jasper.

"Don't you take my baby!" she screamed. "You can't take my baby!" She tried to yank him out of Brad's arms. A staff person appeared immediately and pulled her away. We slipped out the door. Jasper was crying as we stepped into the safety of the lobby.

"She *really* liked you," Brad said, trying to put a positive spin on it.

"No," Jasper said. "I think she thought I was hers."

MY SONS BOUNCED BACK FROM visits much more quickly than I did. I put off going to see Mom for a while after that, and grieved in short but intense bursts when something unlocked the pain. Like Mom's lone sock in a basket in the closet, for example. I recognized it because it was bigger than mine, pilly and worn and missing its mate. She was back for an instant and then gone again. I cried on the floor for a minute. Then it passed.

Another night I heard a song my friend Sandy Lawrence wrote called "When I'm Gone."

You'll wonder why the earth still moves.
You'll wonder how you'll carry on,
But you'll be okay on that first day when I'm gone.

And even though you love me still, you will know where
* you belong.*
Just give it time. We'll both be fine, when I'm gone.

I sobbed so hard I could hardly breathe. I thought about my dad, about how much of his life he'd given to my mother and then lost because of her illness, and about how beautiful and painful it was to see him still hugging and kissing her. I couldn't help despairing. What was the point? She was gone.

THE FOLLOWING JANUARY, SOMETHING SHIFTED. My onetime co-star William Shatner came to Nashville with his wife, Liz. Brad and I went to see his one-man show, *Shatner's World*, at the Tennessee Performing Arts Center.

The Shatners had been friends for years, even before my *Boston Legal* appearance, and we loved our time with them. Bill was vibrant, funny, and honest onstage. He spoke at the end of his performance about the power of saying yes to every facet of life—taking every opportunity, meeting every challenge. I was inspired by that idea, and carried it with me as we went backstage to say hello.

About ten people gathered in Bill's dressing room to congratulate him. In our group was a woman I'd never met before who was guest-starring on the ABC show *Nashville*. I'd had a role on the series for a while, though we'd never overlapped there. I asked her how long she'd lived in Tennessee.

"I came back a couple of years ago to nurse my mother, who had dementia," she said. She told me she had found a profound spiritual connection with her and had a surprising serenity during the last year of her life. "It was very healing," she said. Their time together was different from anything she'd experienced with her mother before. She talked about their energetic communication through music and physical touch. *Huh,* I thought.

We all went to dinner. I sat next to Liz, who asked how my mom was. I never knew how to answer that question. *How is she? Terrible. She's still alive but not. She isn't getting better. She doesn't seem to know us anymore. We're waiting for her to die.*

I didn't say any of these things. "She's fine," I said. "The same."

Liz told me a story about her father, who had passed away seven years previously.

"About a week before he died," she said, "my mother called and said, 'I'm not sure, but it seems like your dad wants to talk to you.'" Liz's father had never been forthcoming with emotion. In fact, she couldn't remember ever hearing him say he loved her. Her mother put him on the phone, and he started talking.

It was a little hard for Liz to understand. But it sounded like, "I love you I love you I love you," over and over and over again. A profound lucidity, perhaps a way of saying goodbye before he died.

I started crying. *I'm missing an opportunity,* I thought. *I need to love my mother in the innocent way my children do. The empathetic way Mom herself has loved people, sometimes total strangers, her whole life. I need to see her as she is, instead of how I want her to be.* Maybe we could find a way to communicate with each other. Maybe then I could let go of the pain. I could be free.

"Yes, go see her," Liz said, wiping away my tears. "Go see your mom."

I got up and walked to Brad, who was on the other side of the room. I sat down on his lap.

"I need to go to New York," I said. He saw my wet cheeks and maybe felt a measure of relief at what seemed to be renewed resolve. I didn't need to explain it much further. He understood.

"Okay," he said.

"Tomorrow."

"Yes."

I GOT ON A PLANE the next day with my brother and my two boys, and we flew north. Something major had shifted in my heart. I felt invigorated, unafraid, open, inspired.

And for the first time in years, my time with Mom didn't hurt.

She was sleeping in a chair, head still bowed, in the living room. Edward was playing "You Are My Sunshine" on his guitar. Gertie sat upright, singing every word in her sweet voice: "You make me happy, when skies are gray!"

"Come *on!*" shouted a man at no one in particular from his wheelchair. Huck and Jasper and I giggled at the strangeness of it all. I shook Mom gently.

"It's me," I said. "It's Kim. A bunch of people are here to see you." When she saw me, her blue eyes opened and she grinned as though I was one of the best surprises of her life. She wasn't a threat anymore, and I could let my defenses down. I took in her joy and accepted it for what it was. Mom was living in the moment. Her lack of self-awareness allowed for a unique kind of peace. I could learn from it.

You are still my teacher.

We sat like that for a while. I rubbed lotion into her hands. Huck and Jasper grabbed my phone and started making videos with Jay. Dad showed me some music therapy techniques he'd learned from a woman named Debby, the new head of the floor. When my mother cried out, "Bah bah bah bah!" as she did often, he mimicked her—syllables, sound qualities, pitch, and volume.

"Bah bah bah bah!" came back at her, mixed like a duet with her voice. The echo seemed to soothe her.

I tried it. It felt silly at first, but I picked it up quickly. As soon as my mother heard herself in my voice, she locked eyes with me. *Connection. We get each other.*

The second part of the technique was to bring down the pitch and volume, and end with a long sigh. Often she would follow and calm herself.

I took a walk with her, fed her, and shared her delight as she rediscovered me every time I left her alone for a moment and then came back. I gave her a big hug when I left.

"I love you, Mom," I said. She smiled and sighed. I left feeling light and happy, with a new understanding. I could choose to see our losses differently.

An acting teacher, Lesly Kahn, once passed along advice attributed to several sources: "Ride the horse in the direction that it's going." *Instead of wishing for things to be different, choose to embrace the life in front of you.* When I let go of my tight grip on expectation, I found I could still have some kind of relationship with my mother. I could share love with her in a beautiful new way.

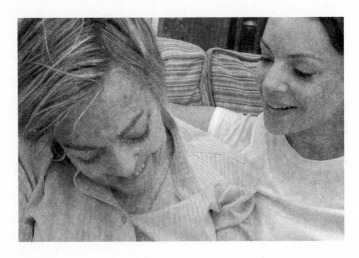

WHEN WE GOT BACK TO Tennessee, my sons proudly showed me the movies they had created while Mom and I had been busy rediscovering our relationship. For years I had felt as if I'd been dipping in and out of a familial war zone. Now that we'd survived, Huck and Jasper had decided to make some comically dark film adaptations. Each one is only a few seconds long. Each was shot using the Action Movie app that lets you create explosive special effects in videos on your iPhone. Jay showed them how that day.

My favorite begins with Mom sitting in the brown comfy chair in her room. She's wearing her pink velour sweatsuit, and her hair is combed assisted-living style. She has a gap in her front teeth where a cap fell off (it would have been too uncomfortable—and unnecessary—to replace it). Dad is on his knees next to her, smiling. I'm on the other side of her, off camera. We're feeding her lunch.

But instantly, *incredibly*, the mood shifts as a gloved hand, wearing a green rectangular watch, enters the frame. Another gloved hand appears and presses a button on a controller. *Clang!* Electric sparks fly. My parents don't notice. The hands disappear. We hear an approaching helicopter. *Thrum thrum thrum thrum.*

Dad carries on, scooping up a spoonful of something orange and mushy. Then there is the chopper, just over his head to the left. Dad doesn't realize it's coming right at him! *In the middle of Mom's bedroom!* They're oblivious to the impending disaster. The helicopter is out of control. It's spinning! It's gonna *crash*! Dad holds the spoon up to Mom's lips. She chews a small bite of sweet potato with her mouth open.

Boom!

The bedroom explodes in a fiery ball! The screen goes black.

(Miraculously, no one is hurt, and life carries on as usual.)

Blessedly, this video makes me laugh as hard as I used to cry.

Dad bet Brad a bottle of wine that he could swim the length of our pond in Tennessee. It was warm that June, as usual, and none of us had ever been in the newly clay-lined, bigger two-acre lake just outside our back door. The water was green, and home to the occasional snapping turtle or snake and many bluegill and bass. It was lovely to paddle across, as we had years before during Festivus, or to cast a fishing lure from the shore for the fun of catch and release. But no one had ever had the courage to take a plunge.

A pair of geese always appeared in March to make a nest on the edge of the water and lay eggs. That summer we watched the three yellow goslings waddling around, learning how to forage. They moved with their parents to the opposite side of the pond when Huck, Jasper, and I joined Dad on the dock in the midafternoon.

It had been a great visit so far—his first solo trip. My father was rested and happy. He had the energy and patience to relax, chat and play with my boys, and get to know them in ways he couldn't before as a hands-on caregiver.

We watched him climb down the ladder from the dock.

"Oh, it's warm!" Dad said as he sank up to his neck. "It's beautiful!" He adjusted his goggles. We held our breath. Would something bite him? Would he get the rare brain-eating amoeba that the media claimed was threatening swimmers in the South in warmer weather? He was unafraid.

"I do this for humanity!" my father cried.

"Really?" I asked.

"No, I do this for the wine," he joked. "If I start to veer off course, give me a shout." And he was off. We watched his calm freestyle. *Stroke, stroke, stroke, breathe.* Within minutes he'd done it—turned that murky pond into a whole new summer joy. We cheered.

The four of us spent the rest of the afternoon floating in life vests and splashing one another, getting our toes nibbled by tiny minnows. My dad introduced us to an adventure we hadn't known existed, right in our own backyard. Most importantly at the time, we felt as if he were ours again.

It had been challenging getting him to leave home long enough for a visit. He was with Mom most days, feeding her and helping with showering and bathroom tasks. He even started working at her residence voluntarily, assisting with training the staff. He gave a class on the technique of "soft eyes," a Zen-like global mindfulness of what's happening in any environment.

Years earlier he'd written an article on how to teach children to protect themselves, and interviewed a martial arts expert about how kids and others could expand their senses to anticipate danger. Dad thought that educating the employees of the dementia-care floor on the practice might help them keep tabs on many residents at once, allowing them to be aware, for example, that someone all the way across the room might fall.

My father had become a part of the fabric of Mom's new home, making friends, learning names, and listening to stories, helping in whatever way he could every time he was there. He did this because he appreciated the unique challenges in a community like this, and the people who were responsible for handling them. And also because he believed that his continued involvement would ensure that my mother would get the best possible care. He still loved her deeply. He kissed and hugged her, and danced with his arms around her waist to help hold her up. He sang her favorite songs.

"I'm so glad I married you," he said to her during every visit. "And I'm so glad you didn't marry that Bill guy," Mom's boyfriend before she met Dad. Sometimes she responded with a smile or a laugh, though it didn't really seem as if she was processing what he was saying.

So it took me by surprise when he made a confession to me privately that summer in Tennessee: He wanted to find a compatible partner to spend the rest of his life with. He missed having someone.

"Actually," he said, "I've already been on a few dates with women."

Oh, God, I thought. I sat opposite him at the kitchen table in the cabin, suddenly very uncomfortable. We were alone in the house, and that was probably why he'd brought it up. I shifted in my seat and tried to take in what he was saying. But this was not what I wanted to hear. *Mom is still alive,* I thought. *You are still married.*

"I'm just starting to meet people," he went on. "And I want to have your blessing."

He told me he'd recently encountered a classmate at his college reunion in a similar situation. The man had fallen in love with a woman while his dementia-ridden wife was still living with him. The wife was completely dependent and mostly unaware of anything, as Mom was. He told my father the success of the new relationship depended largely on family support.

"You have it," I told my dad, not knowing if I meant it. "I want you to do what you need to do to be happy." Truthfully, though, I was dying for the conversation to be over. I added, "Maybe I don't need to hear details unless it gets really serious."

It was just too painful to think about at first. Part of me felt as if I owed it to my mother not to support my dad in this new endeavor, although from a logical standpoint in more lucid times, I supposed she would have been okay with it.

She wouldn't have wanted him to be unhappily alone. I didn't know for sure, though, since they'd never discussed the possibility of such a scenario.

Could Dad's dating life get in the way of his remaining duties as my mother's husband? Why wasn't he content with getting to know his grandkids and having adventures in our backyard? We'd just gotten him back. And what kind of person would be willing to be with a man who already had a wife?

I selfishly hoped he wouldn't find anyone.

As the months passed, his dating life started to feel like the elephant in the room. Dad was able to discuss it openly with Ashley and her husband, Neal—they celebrated the fact that he was meeting people and cultivating relationships. But Jay, Brad, and I had a harder time embracing it. Dad and I had always been close, able to discuss anything. Now I'd asked him not to share details of a big part of his life with me. I wanted to know, but at the same time I felt uneasy every time he tried to talk about it. I am my mother's daughter.

"I had a nice evening last night," he'd say over the phone cryptically. "With ... somebody that we don't need to talk about if you don't want to but if you do let me know." *Ugh*. He was dying to tell me. While he was trying to be respectful, his dancing around it made me feel even more awkward.

"That's great!" I'd say as cheerfully as possible, and promptly change the subject.

One friend who'd had parents in a similar situation told

me, "People are meant to be together. Your dad shouldn't have to be alone if he doesn't want to be."

Many others agreed. "Good for him," they said.

But some people pointed out, "The vows say 'in sickness and in health' and 'until death do us part.'" They were encouraging me to nudge my father away from this path. "This is the 'in sickness' part," they said. "Don't just sign off on this."

One of those people had been married for years to someone who had divorced her first spouse, and it made me think.

Would we have been more able to accept Dad's dating if he had divorced my mom? After she bit him for the first time, maybe, or almost pushed him down the stairs? My father had stuck by my mother and been loyal to a fault. He still loved her. And yet he was declaring that he also needed companionship and intellectual and emotional stimulation. The more I wrestled with it, the more I found myself starting to defend his choices, even as I didn't want to know about them.

Brad played devil's advocate, joking with me one day after I told him about a particularly awkward phone call with my father, "Your mother would be rolling over in her grave right now—if she were dead."

I found the irony very funny.

She wasn't dead, of course. If she were, I could look up into the starry night sky and imagine her whole and vibrant again, my guardian angel. I could let her go. We could move on. Would it then be easier for me to let my father go, too?

I thought back to when I was younger, and the first time I left my parents to go to kindergarten, to date boys I liked, to travel to a college far from home, to move to California, to manage my own finances, to marry. To do something they didn't necessarily approve of. Every departure of mine was as it should have been. I was finding my own way.

I thought about my own kids. I loved inhaling the smell of Jasper's hair as I kissed him in his sleep after a long summer day of play—the scent a perfect mixture of dirt, sunscreen, and sweet cookie. I loved holding up Huck's tiny palm to my own.

"One day your hands will be bigger than mine," I'd tell him. "And you'll look down at me and say, 'Hi, Mom.'" He'd giggle at my mock-deep voice and then I'd nibble his neck.

They'd already left me for their first days of school. And I'd left them, too, to go to work, to vacation, to take respite time from parenting. Now I usually got a "See ya—love ya!" and a quick hug. No more little arms wrapped around my pant leg as they begged me not to leave. No more crocodile tears. We would have many more goodbyes between us.

This is the arc of a family. Over the years, there are a series of arrivals and departures. And in the midst of that, part of the challenge is encouraging the people we love to become independent, and to love them as they are. Dad deserved to be happy the way he wanted to be. Realistically, I hadn't ever "had him back." He wasn't ever mine to have. I needed to let him go, as he had let me go. I needed to let him jump into the water.

I allowed myself a passing flash of a thought: *Maybe Dad will meet someone that I'll love, too.*

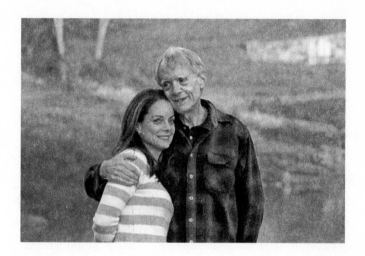

I SUMMONED ENOUGH COURAGE ONE day to ask him about a woman I knew he'd been dating for a couple of months. He was startled by my question and my willingness to talk about it. To my surprise, he didn't say much. Right after we got off the phone, though, he sent me an email.

Before he could tell me more about her, he wrote, he wanted me to do something. "Please read a little of the first chapter of a book called *In Lieu of Flowers*. This style of writing matches what you were talking about, what you'd like for your book." *Huh. Okay.*

I was beginning to think about writing a book about this experience. I'd gotten some attention for a magazine piece I'd written, and the response to it made me realize I had an opportunity to help people by sharing my story. I was reading everything I could to see how others like me had told their stories. I didn't know why Dad's request took priority over my question about his dating life, but I was happy to put off the other conversation. Immediately I found and read the first chapter of *In Lieu of Flowers: A Conversation for the Living*, by Nancy Howard Cobb. I discovered that it was a book about grief, love, and loss. Both of the author's parents had had dementia.

"My parents are my guideposts," she writes. "Losing them made me a bit braver about saying what needs to be said, to people who are dying, to people who are grieving, to people who are afraid to talk at all. . . . If you give yourself permission to talk about your experience, you'll find that other people will want to talk about theirs."

I wrote my father back right away.

"I love the writing in this book," I said. "She is terrific."

She, he told me then, was the woman he'd recently become very involved with. I'd known nothing about her. They'd been introduced via email through a mutual friend. They met for the first time at an Italian restaurant near Grand Central Station in New York, and talked and laughed for such a long time that my father was uncharacteristically late for an appointment. They found common ground about growing up as only children, caregiving, and writing. On their second date, they were so engrossed in each other that the waitress came over to their table and told them she'd never seen a couple so "romantic."

My father's way of initially introducing his new partner was a good idea. I already liked Nancy Cobb as a writer. About two months later, we met in person.

I was nervous, and as I rode the elevator up to her Manhattan apartment, I was resolved to step cautiously into this new territory. But all of my hesitations dissipated when Nancy opened the door and hugged me tightly. She stepped back, and I noticed that her bright hazel eyes were tearing up.

"I want you to know, I honor you," she said as she held me by both shoulders. "And I honor your mom. And I know this is hard."

She led me past my father, who seemed to be giddy. He looked younger, cooler. Handsome. He was wearing properly fitted trousers maybe for the first time in his life, and a classy rose-colored button-down shirt I'd never seen before. Nancy and I sat together on her couch with glasses of wine in front of some snacks she'd laid out. Almost immediately we began talking and laughing like old friends.

Later, as my dad and I left to go to dinner alone, they kissed each other goodbye. I had to look away. It was the first time I'd ever seen my father be affectionate in that way with another woman, and it tugged at my heart. Nevertheless, I was encouraged. *She actually seems great.*

LATER THAT SUMMER, I GOT a call from Dad. He'd been diagnosed with stage 1 prostate cancer.

"This is eminently treatable," he insisted on the phone. He would receive low-level radiation treatments weekdays in fifteen-minute sessions, close to his home, and be finished in about two months. There would be minimal side effects—"probably," he told me.

I asked him if he needed me to come to New York. He said that Jay was going to be with him for a few days, and other than that, with Nancy's help, he'd be fine. I largely put it out of my mind.

In September I hosted a baby shower for my sister. Ashley was the last sibling in the family to have a child, and she'd shared with me over the months that she was grieving not having Mom there for her pregnancy and early motherhood.

She told me she'd visited our mother and struggled to tell her that a new grandchild was on the way. She wanted to feel Mom's hand on her belly, to celebrate what was happening. *You were pregnant with me and now I'm pregnant with him,* she thought. A mother-daughter milestone. She wanted a photo of the moment.

But Mom wasn't cooperating. She kept her hands curled up next to her and opened her mouth to bite my sister's finger every time she tried to move one of Mom's arms away from her body. Finally, as my mother started to drift off to sleep, her hand twitched out within reach. Ash grabbed it and slapped it onto her stomach. She tossed her phone to an aide to get the picture. It was a terrible memento. She left feeling silly and awful.

"I so badly wanted her to register what was happening,"

Ash told me. "But she couldn't. She just slumped there. She missed it."

I wanted to make up for the family celebration she hadn't had, to spoil her. I also loved any excuse to spend some time with her. We met up in California with nine of her girlfriends for a relaxed spa-type weekend. Her friends and I hired a team of women to offer reflexology and henna tattoos, and a chef to cook for us, and we spent two days swimming, napping, hiking, eating, and talking about men, babies, labor, parents, books, movies, and everything else we could think of.

Before the weekend began, Ashley handed me a present that I opened privately, in my bedroom. I lifted the lid on the square brown box and saw a necklace. It was Mom's. It brought back a flood of memories.

I took her out one day as something to do. Were we in LA? We found a shop that offered custom-made charm jewelry, and I helped her pick out a silver rectangular piece on which they imprinted Huck's name and a bronze piece for Jasper's name. We chose a tiny heart charm to go with it, but Mom wanted to add more. A dragonfly. She hadn't liked the simple chain I picked for some reason—was it too short around her neck? When we got back to the house, Dad took the charms off for her and threaded them together with a longer thin silver cable from another necklace she owned. She put it on. We laughed as she hugged me while she bounced up and down, awkward but endearing. The gift was her prized possession for a while.

I'd forgotten all about it. I asked my sister where it had been.

"Nancy found it," Ashley said. "It was in a box in Mom's chest of drawers." Dad had long delayed sorting through the jewelry, trinkets, Christmas pins, hats, socks, and other small but powerful reminders of Mom. Most of her favorites had gone with her to her new home. Dad asked Nancy to sift through what was left and put all the pieces on display so Ashley could choose what the three of us might like to keep.

My heart ached, and again I laughed at the irony of how the necklace came to be back in my hands.

AFTER EVERYONE LEFT THE BABY shower, Ash and Neal and Brad and I went out to dinner. We had a great night, catching up and reliving the best moments of the weekend. It was almost eleven as we drove back to our house in separate cars. My phone rang, but I didn't hear it and it went to voicemail. I listened to it a minute later. It was Neal, trying to sound calm.

"Please call your sister as soon as you get this."

She'd received a message from the assisted-living facility. Our mother had had a seizure—a dangerously long one, maybe four minutes. Afterward she was unresponsive. An aide called an ambulance, and they took her to the hospital. Now the staff member who'd accompanied her needed to leave. He was supposed to have gone home a couple of hours earlier.

No one had been able to reach my dad since the incident. I had an email in my inbox from Debby, saying my father wasn't answering calls, texts, or email. They also couldn't reach Sheelah, his emergency contact. The staff needed to know what we wanted them to do. Mom was stable and asleep. Did we want to hire someone to stay with her or allow her to be alone?

From three thousand miles away, we didn't know. Was she in danger of hurting herself? Falling out of bed? Pulling out an IV?

Ash and I sat on the bed talking it through, communicating with Debby, who was at home, all of us trying to get an accurate picture of what was going on. Meanwhile, what had happened to Dad? I had a slight fear he was in some trouble, but my overwhelming sense was that it was something else.

"He's with his girlfriend!" I moaned to my sister more than once. "This is not okay. If he is going to go off somewhere with her, he needs to leave his phone on, leave proper backup information. This is completely irresponsible." I felt as if we were talking about two teenagers. I pictured Dad and Nancy slumbering together somewhere, oblivious. All of the fears and resentments I'd had in the beginning came flooding back.

Eventually, kind and generous Debby got out of bed and drove forty-five minutes to the hospital to see for herself how our mother was doing. She sat by Mom's bedside until morning. Ashley and I each had a sleepless night, constantly rolling over in our beds to check our phones. We'd left messages everywhere—for Sheelah, for Dad, for Nancy, and even for Nancy's daughter Leland.

Sheelah was the first to respond in the morning. She went to my father's house and rang the doorbell. He answered cheerfully. He was alone. He was finishing up breakfast and reading a newspaper.

He'd had his first radiation treatment the day before and was exhausted, as much from the reality of his cancer as the treatment itself. He'd slept much more heavily than he'd expected. His cell had been next to him on a bedside table, set as always on vibrate. But he had been so out of it that he hadn't even heard any of the calls on it or the house phone.

Now he rushed to the hospital to be by my mother's side. And when Nancy found out, she canceled her meetings in Manhattan to be there for Dad. It took him two days to get my mother out of the hospital because of various tests and consultations. It seemed to all of us like overkill for someone with her disease.

My father continued with his treatments over the next two months, and Nancy became more vigilant. She made sure he ate, drank the liter of water prescribed before radiation every day, and got rest. She listened to him, laughed with him, and helped him restore his battered sense of humor. I went from resenting her the night we couldn't reach him to feeling profoundly grateful that Dad had someone he loved by his side.

. . .

THE HOSPITAL VISIT TAUGHT US it was time to update my mother's advance directives. Dad filled out a revised New York State MOLST form (Medical Orders for Life-Sustaining Treatment). As he had in the past, he checked the "do not resuscitate," or DNR, box, and another box for "comfort measures only," including the offer of food and fluids by mouth and meds to relieve pain and suffering. He vetoed several interventions, such as further trips to the hospital, unless pain for severe symptoms couldn't otherwise be controlled. He asked to be consulted before any antibiotic use.

After the seizure, which showed the progression of her condition, she qualified for hospice care, a Medicare-backed end-of-life program focused on minimizing pain and discomfort. She was supplied with a new hospital bed and a high-backed wheelchair, an oxygen tank in case she needed it, and all incontinence supplies formerly paid for by my father. A one-on-one nurse supplemented the staff on her floor for four hours a day, five days a week. Though the term *hospice* conjured up a sickening reality for me that we were in the last phase of Mom's disease, I was nevertheless grateful that her care was tailored specifically to her needs.

THE NEXT TIME I SAW Nancy, a month later in New York, she and my dad and I went to dinner. I sat between them as we rode to the restaurant in a cab. Nancy had recently visited Mom for the first time. She was surprised at how painful it was for her to see her partner's wife in that state. But they laughed together and held hands.

"It's not fair," Nancy told me in the car. She was crying. "It's not fair, that she's in there and I'm out here with your father." She shrugged, and then shook her head, looking out the window. I admired her vulnerability and courage to talk about what we were all thinking but not saying.

"Everyone's been focused on Dad and us kids," I said. "What's this like for you?"

"It's hard," she said, and paused to think for a moment. "But I often find that messy, complicated situations bring people closer than we would be otherwise. Your mother is a part of my life now. And she always will be. I am your ally, and hers."

THE GARDEN AT BARBETTA, A restaurant on West Forty-sixth Street, was lush and cozy. We sat at a table near the back wall. Nancy and my father had separately dined there in the 1970s. Our cheeky Italian waiter said he remembered Dad from decades ago.

"You were with a different woman then, no?" he said.

The fact that this stranger somehow picked up on that truth, even if he was just guessing, sent us into hearty, healing laughter.

Later, my new ally and I stole away to the bathroom together. Both of us sensed we needed to talk privately, girl to girl.

"Thank you," I told her as we stood beside the sink in the small space. "You know, the idea of my dad dating was . . ." I took a half step back and crossed my index fingers in the air as if warding away an evil spirit. The symbol seemed clearer than the words I had to finish the sentence. Nancy nodded and laughed. I took a deep breath.

"But if I could have imagined the ideal person for him now, it would have been you," I said. "I am so grateful."

We hugged. I meant it.

thought this story would end with Mom's death.

She didn't die.

In fact, she rallied. She had no further seizures. Her vital signs were stable. Her blood pressure was normal, her heart strong. She fared so well with hospice care that it was discontinued after six months, just a few weeks before Easter.

One of the early days after the hospital visit, my father met with a Reiki therapist on the couch outside my mom's room. Dad asked her how his wife had reacted to the treatment she'd just performed, a kind of laying on of hands.

"I don't know," the woman said, looking troubled. "Linda wasn't very responsive. It's almost as though she doesn't have a soul."

She appeared to regret her words as soon as they'd left her mouth. But I was infuriated when I heard the story. How dare this stranger suggest dementia had robbed my mother of her eternal spirit, along with everything else? Just because she wasn't able to perceive Mom's soul didn't mean it wasn't there.

Or did it?

I was embarrassed to admit that I understood what she meant. Mom's eyes—"the windows to the soul"—were often vacant now. I believed that we each had a consciousness, or self, that transcended our earthly bodies. I had faith that if my mother died, her spirit would survive. But now I started to wonder, where was that soul in this purgatory of dementia? Sleeping? Awake and vibrant in ways I couldn't see? What happens to consciousness when the brain deteriorates?

Mom used to embrace the possibility of miracles, but she had a harder time believing in God. She wanted to, and envied people who did. She celebrated the divine gifts of family, laughter, mystery, discovery, science, love. But not the afterlife.

"I just don't know if I buy it," she would say. I respected her honesty.

AS HER DISEASE PROGRESSED, I sometimes wondered if PPA could be a cosmic lesson crafted just for her, a weakening of her rational mind so she could let go and discover what essential truths lay beyond reason. I wondered why she was still alive, three years after being moved to the dementia-care community, when her doctors had pointed to statistics suggesting that she'd already outlived many with her condition. Maybe she was ready to die but was afraid. Maybe she was holding on for something. Maybe I could help.

During a visit, I asked my father to leave Mom and me alone in her bedroom. She was in her wheelchair, head down, hands in her lap. I knelt in front of her to make eye contact.

"Mom," I said, holding on to her knees. "Many, many people love you deeply. Me especially." Her eyes opened wider, as they often did when someone spoke to her, and she seemed to look at me in wonder.

"We will always love you and celebrate you. No matter what." Her gaze drifted to the side as though she was processing what I was saying. I continued.

"I was wondering," I said. "Are you ready to leave this place?" She straightened up, then glanced out the window and back to me, as though she thought she was supposed to do something but couldn't understand the directions. I realized I had to be more specific.

"What I mean, Mom," I said, "is that when you are ready to leave this world, it's all right. We'll be okay. And I believe that you'll be okay, too." She took a deep breath and sighed. A tear rolled down her cheek. Was she understanding me?

"This has been hard," I said, trying to mirror what I guessed she felt. I held her wrinkled, bony hand in mine, waiting, giving myself time to settle on what I had to say. And then I went on.

"I believe, Mom, that when you're done here, when

you're ready to be free of this body, that you are gonna get to dance. And party. And fly. And be healed." She gazed above my head, as though something amazing had just caught her attention. A vision? An angel? Or just a spot of dirt? I glanced behind me. Nothing but a white wall.

I sang one of her favorite songs. She still seemed to be uplifted by music.

"Amazing grace, how sweet the sound . . ." She stared above me for the length of the song. I'd not seen her this alert in a long time. I had more to tell her. I took another deep breath.

"I believe that God loves you, Mom," I said. "And that when you die, your soul will live on. I believe that you'll go to heaven." And my mother looked right at me, fully alert, and said the first clear sentence I'd heard from her in more than a year.

"No, I won't."

The disappointment that my mother hadn't embraced a new belief or answered my larger "why" question paralleled my delight over getting a rare glimpse of lucid, authentic Mom. Part of her was still in there.

She's not ready to die yet.

I TRIED TO CONNECT WITH her again when I went to see her next. This time I came with something I knew she used to believe in: bourbon. Brad had given me an appreciation for what was once Mom's beverage of choice.

He told me that bourbon is like a time machine. The final result is a combination of factors. Each batch is different and contains memories, of the crop that year and the quality of the grains. Bourbon is a different kind of time machine for me. One sniff takes me back to my childhood. Maybe it would do the same for Mom. *She deserves a little party,* I thought.

So I snuck a silver flask full of Evan Williams 1783 onto the fifth floor. Debby probably would've let me bring it in openly, but I didn't want to ask. *Besides,* I thought, *Mom would appreciate a covert operation.* Brad chose Evan Williams for me because it was the same company that made Heaven Hill—the cheapest bourbon available to my parents when I was a kid. This version would possibly be the best she'd ever tasted.

I didn't know if it would interfere with her current meds, so I decided to pour only a few drops onto a spoon. Neat—no water, no ice, no soda. First I held it up to her nose. Bourbon sometimes burned my nostrils when I tipped my nose into a glass. I wondered if it would do the same for her on the spoon. Dementia patients often lose their sense of smell. She didn't react.

Bourbon usually singed the tip of my tongue when I drank it. It made my eyes water. Mom used to have it diluted with ice every night. Would she spit it out now or want more? I was a little nervous as I brought it to her lips. She opened her mouth, as she did anytime something was put in front of it, and I tilted the caramel-colored liquid onto her tongue. I waited.

Nothing. It was as though I'd given her a sip of water. The drink puddled in her mouth, and eventually she must have swallowed it because it didn't dribble back out again. She stared straight ahead without any reaction.

Instead of embracing New Mom the way I'd been learning to do, I went home this time feeling sad. Maybe we would never reconnect again in a way I could understand. And my questions remained: Why was she still here? Sometimes lucid but often not? What was the larger spiritual lesson in all of this? What was I supposed to do now?

When I told my therapist, Karen, about the bourbon experiment, the heaven conversation and Mom's response, and my questions as to the whereabouts of her soul, she told me, "Consciousness is there in ways you can't understand or explain the way your ego wants to." She added that I was focusing on the wrong thing.

"These questions are about you, not her," she told me in her no-nonsense way. "You're projecting what you want to see onto your mother. The pain, the joy, the connection or lack of connection—all of it."

It's what many of us do. "Linda was happy today," her caregivers say. Or "I think she missed you."

"Your mom seems calm," Dad reports after a visit.

"Mom was really attentive," I tell Dad after our God talk. To think so makes me feel better. And when I guess that she isn't clued in with me, I feel sad. But again, I could choose to project something else.

"Here is your work," Karen said. "Don't look at what you're not getting from your mother. Look at what you are getting." It was a lesson I thought I'd already learned. But it was time to delve deeper.

THIS IS WHAT I CAME up with: My mother is not only presenting me an opportunity to love unconditionally, she's also allowing me to practice being comfortable with what is uncomfortable. To grieve and also embrace what is broken. To know that some days I can receive who my mother is now and some days I struggle with it. To allow that two opposing thoughts may exist in my head at the same time.

I want things to be the way they were, and I am relieved that they never will be again. I regret I didn't feel more acceptance from my mother at times in my life, and I'm grateful for the lesson she is giving me now in accepting myself. Jay put it this way: "Letting go of what she used to be has been the hardest act, and yet the most liberating."

This emotional clash within me feels like the eagle pose in yoga. You wrap one bent knee around the other and hook your foot on the back of your standing leg. Then you twist your arms in a similar fashion and bring your hands together in front of your face. Oxygen and circulation are limited. But still, you try to breathe and avoid falling. As you stare at your sweaty self in the mirror, you attempt to smile and stay present, even when you want to quit. Many days I see my red-faced struggling self in the mirror, and I don't feel like the regal bird this pose is named for. But some days I kind of do. I accept this.

My dad told us a story about running a strange article in *Omni* magazine, where he was the editor in the 1980s. It was about a wild plan from a scientist who suggested that someday we might send a flotilla of insulated spaceships to the sun to collect its plasma and truck it back to Earth. It would provide all of our energy needs. The topic was typical of the publication, a mixture of science and science fiction. An *Omni* staffer called a physicist at Princeton to weigh in and provide balance. What he said at first wasn't surprising: "It's not gonna happen."

But then he went on: "What's going to happen will be much more fantastic than that." It was a line my father quoted often as we were growing up, and it became the core of a kind of optimistic surrender to what we couldn't know. In accepting our limited wisdom, we allow for infinite possibility.

NANCY SENT ME SOME HELPFUL words one day after I told her that I was struggling with writing a difficult chapter in this book. They were from the Leonard Cohen song "Anthem":

Ring the bells that still can ring.
Forget your perfect offering.
There is a crack in everything.
That's how the light gets in.

The lyrics became *my* anthem as I sought to make sense of what's happened to my mother, my family, and me. Many other people, some I hardly or never knew, aided my quest.

I learned that even near death, some people with dementia can communicate their love. I was able to find new ways to connect with my mother. Then I learned that the messages I got from her followed no deathbed script, suggested no happy or sad ending. I realized that every time I cast my mother in some sort of role—New Mom, Mom headed for heaven, Mom with no soul—real life intruded to say, *You can't really know her, can you?*

She's more of a puzzle now than she was when I began writing this book. But lately, just when I think I've lost her, I find her again in small things and brief moments. They deepen the mystery, and feel something like miracles.

IT WAS DURING A TALK with Veronique at the Fox Foundation that I first learned how Mom attached gold paper clips to mailings for people she wanted to make feel special. After I spoke with her, I sat writing for a couple of hours, thinking about the significance of this simple tool, meant to hold things together. Finally I got up to stretch and get a drink in the pantry off our kitchen. Something flashed at me from the middle of the floor: a gold paper clip.

We use silver paper clips. Red and blue and green and yellow paper clips. Never gold. I'm sure we probably had a few in the house, perhaps from a Fox Foundation mailing. Veronique told me that Mom's gold-clip initiative had become a tradition. But what brought it to the pantry on that particular day? I showed it to Huck, who had no idea that it carried deep meaning to Mom, and now to me.

"Oh, yeah," he said, "I found that in the bag"—an old recycling sack hanging on the back of a chair in the kitchen. Of course it could have been just a coincidence. But I took it as a sign from my mother to me. We were still connected by a bond as enduring as precious metal, but much more fantastic than that.

A couple of months later, I found another gold paper clip, and then about a month later, another. Sure, I was looking harder for them, but each showed up somewhere it wasn't supposed to be: on the floor under a dining table in a friend's house, in the little cup holder of a treadmill. I found the most ornate gold paper clip I have ever seen in the back of my car, under the seat. It looked like an elaborate treble clef.

"Oh, yeah," Huck said. "I got that from my music teacher last year." But I took comfort from what I chose to believe. It was left behind to travel with me.

One night in the car on the way home from a great dinner in downtown Nashville, I was telling my friends Tracie and Missy about the wondrous paper clip sightings.

"I'm calling it a God wink," I said. "It's as if God is winking at me and saying, *I'm here. And there is more going on than you realize.*" I remembered that there had been other God winks in my life: my mother spewing Grandpa's colorful profanity at the moment my eight-year-old self was asking him for help. The woman waiting for me in the hospital chapel around the corner from my cousin's room right after he died. And now the gorgeous gold clef at my side in the center console of my car.

"Yes! A God wink!" my friends cheered.

And at that moment we rounded a curve and our headlights illuminated an albino deer staring at us on the side of the road. Ever since I had moved to Nashville, I'd assumed that stories about this regal creature were fables. By some estimates there are only a few dozen of them in Tennessee, and most residents would be lucky to see even one. But there it stood, still and majestic, pure white, a giant rack on its head. We gasped and reached out for one another. *Are we all seeing this?* There was no doubt for any of us that this was an exclamation mark on our conversation.

That is where the light gets in.

MOM WAS GETTING HER NAILS done when Huck and I arrived for a visit recently. This activity is a challenge because it's hard for her to sit still. The technician was a master at it. He wore rubber gloves and worked with speed and precision. He was blowing warm air on my mother's right hand when we sat down with her.

"She's dry," he said. "I'll come back for the other hand in a bit so you have time to visit."

"Hi, Nana," Huck said. Mom saw him and sighed. She stared at the carpet. "Hi, Nana," he repeated, not giving up.

We wheeled her into the dining room and placed her in front of a helping of salad, a hard-boiled egg that slipped around the plate, and some soup. I fed her while Huck sat next to me making more special-effects disaster videos, this time about giant floods and sinkholes stealing the meal. Mom was quiet.

She'd had good days recently, Debby told me. During lunch a couple of weeks earlier, the staff struggled to maneuver several wheelchairs around in a small space. Suddenly Debby felt a kick on her backside. She turned around and saw my mom.

"Sorry, Linda!" she said. Debby is the kind of person who apologizes when someone bumps into her. My mother was stone-faced. Debby turned away. She felt another kick. She whirled again and saw Mom's leg stretched out in front of her as far as it could reach from the wheelchair.

"Wait . . . did you just kick me? In the butt?"

My mother's mouth opened wide. She cackled.

She'd pulled off a prank. A joke! Even better, her laughter was contagious. The staff in the kitchen cracked up, and so did Debby. She told me it's rare to find a dementia patient with some sense of humor still intact.

But during our visit that day in the kitchen, Mom was withdrawn and sleepy. I accepted her as she was, disconnected from Huck and me. I didn't work overtime to try to draw her out.

I observed my sadness, and my conflicted feelings about the lunch she ate robotically, bite by bite, whenever I displayed a morsel of something in front of her mouth. My mom appeared to be no more hungry than she was aware of us. *Am I force-feeding her?* In a small act of protest, I offered her only half of the meal, then cleared the dishes. I gave her a big hug and kissed her on the cheek.

"I love you, Mom," I said. She didn't respond.

As my son and I walked down the hall toward the exit, we were wondering the same thing.

Huck said, "How's your book gonna end?"

ON A WARM DAY IN California, I took the boys to the beach. I sat on the sand as they ran in and out of the surf. The sun was on its way down into the Pacific, and I shielded my eyes from the glare. For a while Huck and Jasper hauled bushels of seaweed, rocks, and shells out of the water, and made a pile that looked like giant slimy sea spaghetti.

"I'm collecting evidence!" Huck yelled when I asked what he was doing. The more they played, the wetter they got.

"Come in with us!" Jasper called to me.

I hesitated. *It sure is cozy here on this towel. I'm dry. I'm warm. I'm happy watching.*

But then, in a big *duh, aha* moment, I knew what I had to do.

My bare feet navigated through the little wet pebbles and sand crabs so I could grab a four-foot-long hunk of kelp and drag it out of the water. *Evidence.*

Huck and I got the boogie boards and strapped the Velcro bracelets around our wrists so we wouldn't lose them. Jasper took off up and down the beach, flapping his arms to make dragon wings. Huck and I turned and held up our boards like shields against the waves. We pushed back each time one hit, and then forged ahead. Finally waist-deep, I dove in headfirst. Coming up for air, I sucked in my breath and felt that familiar cold shock. My ears ached as the wind whipped past and the salt stung my eyes. Almost immediately, it was invigorating. *This is Mom,* I thought. *Alive in me.*

The vibrant end-of-day light made me squint, and I silently thanked my mother for this adventure. Huck and I turned around to face the shore. We caught a wave on the second try, and screamed in delight as we rode it the whole way in.

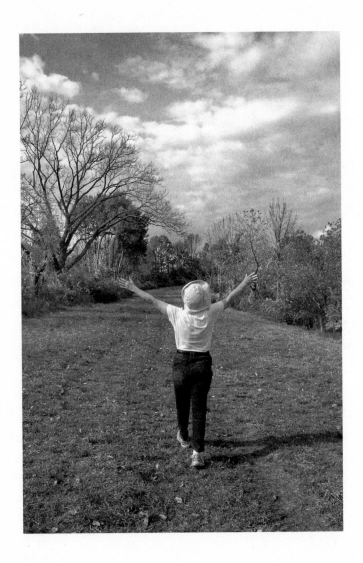

RESOURCES

What would Mom say if she were well and could understand this book?

She was hesitant at first about revealing her dementia. But eventually she told many people and drew comfort from their support. I think if she'd been able, she would have followed Michael J. Fox's example by going public, making a mission of shattering taboos, and raising money for research.

She might have objected that this memoir didn't adequately portray the horror of her condition. *It was more shit in a bucket than where the light gets in,* she might have said. But almost above all, she would've demanded that we acknowledge the many mistakes we made, and insisted that I provide you with access to key resources we wish we had discovered years ago. So, in a way, all of what follows is from my mother to you. (All links referenced in this section can be easily accessed through my website, www.wherethelightgetsinbook.com.)

How Big Is the Threat of Dementia?

The projections are alarming. By 2025, the number of people age sixty-five and older with Alzheimer's disease will reach more than seven million in the US. Females in their sixties are about twice as likely to develop AD sometime in their lives as they are to get breast cancer. These patients of the future will face daunting expenses. Already today, end-of-life health-care costs for people with dementia are substantially larger than those for cancer or heart disease. Yet, in spite of these numbers, funding support for essential research lags.

For more facts and figures, see: http://www.alz.org /news_and_events_women_in_their_60s.asp; http://annals .org/article.aspx?articleid=2466364; http://report.nih.gov /PFSummaryTable.aspx.

What Can You Do to Help?

Get involved. Mom would have asked you to donate money (generously) to an established nonprofit organization like the three listed below. Become an advocate on behalf of the millions of people like my mother who cannot speak out for themselves. Spread information about the stats above (on social media, letters to editors and Washington representatives, one-to-one conversations ...) that will be news to many. Donate online at the Alzheimer's Association (http://www.alz .org/join_the_cause_donate.asp); the Lewy Body Association (http://www.lbda.org/donate); or the Association for Frontotemporal Dementia (http://www.theaftd.org/get-involved /ways-to-give).

How Do You Know If You or Someone You Love Has Dementia?

Everyone in my family and many friends have asked this question since Mom's diagnosis. We've found this link, about normal aging versus Alzheimer's, to be reassuring: www.alz .org/alzheimers_disease_10_signs_of_alzheimers.asp#signs.

But if your answers don't dispel your concerns, your next step might be to check in with a physician.

Where Can You Get a Reliable Diagnosis?

Mom's internist was the first to give her a few simple tests. Struggling with them didn't mean she had dementia. It took many more hours of testing and examinations to zero in on a likely reason for her symptoms and exclude other possible causes. Start here to get the basics and find a physician near you: www.alz.org/alzheimers_disease_diagnosis.asp.

This overview summarizes major types of dementia, including primary progressive aphasia (under the general category of frontotemporal dementia): www.alz.org/professionals _and_researchers_13507.asp.

Specifically for information about PPA, go to the place where it was named in the 1980s, at Northwestern University: http://brain.northwestern.edu/dementia/ppa/.

Look here to explore symptoms and causes (including the finding that in some cases, PPA is caused by Alzheimer's disease): http://brain.northwestern.edu/dementia/ppa/signs .html.

This site points out that some dementias are reversible: https://caregiver.org/diagnosing-dementia.

And this 2013 medical journal article is about how some conditions mimic Alzheimer's. It's not a quick read, so maybe pass it on to your physician: http://www.ncbi.nlm.nih.gov /pmc/articles/PMC3725959.

How Could Stigma Hurt You?

The secrecy we sought was a feverish side effect of Mom's dementia in the early months after her diagnosis. We've learned it's not an uncommon obsession, particularly among comparatively young people like her. And it's understandable. If she'd been worn down by cancer or heart disease, it might have been easier to expect support from an employer and time off for a treatment likely to succeed. Once cancer itself was unmentionable. Until the 1970s, doctors often hid findings of malignancy from patients because tumors were shrouded in stigma.

More than half a century later, dementia attacked my mother's voice, and shame silenced her from saying the disease's name to friends and her employer for more than a year. Those twelve months of untold pain got us off to a bad start when concealing the truth kept us from receiving expert advice about how to deal with a family disaster. This survey published in 2012 suggests that about a quarter of respondents with dementia conceal or hide their diagnosis: www.alz.org /documents_custom/world_report_2012_final.pdf.

How Can You Get Free, Individualized Help from Actual People?

Call the Alzheimer's Association 24/7 help line at 800-272-3900. You will be transferred automatically to a local chapter of the Chicago-based organization. This is one of the best all-around services for patients and caregivers, fielding questions and referring callers to national and local resources. The association's website, www.alz.org, also maintains a broad menu of helpful information on all of the dozens of kinds of dementia.

If the diagnosis is frontotemporal dementia (FTD), the Association for Frontotemporal Degeneration (AFTD) is reachable through its help line, 866-507-7222. You can find general information from the AFTD site: www.theaftd.org/life-with -ftd/newly-diagnosed. From there you can link to a helpful online pamphlet called *The Doctor Thinks It's FTD. Now What?*

What Resources Are Tailored Specifically for Caregivers?

Here is where to find up-to-date information about online communities, tools for navigating care, a stress check, books, a care-team calendar, communication, and more: www.alz .org/care/.

Look at this set of specific steps to take if you're just beginning to take care of someone else: www.caregiveraction .com/i-just-realized-im-family-caregiver-now-0.

The same site has ideas for long-term caregivers, people with the double burden of taking care of someone while holding a job or living far away from patients.

If, like us, your family members live in separate states, here's a guide to long-distance caregiving: https://caregiver .org/sites/caregiver.org/files/pdfs/LongDistanceCG_Hand book_2014.pdf.

And this online handbook is a guide to finding, evaluating, and paying for respite care—time off for caregivers: http:// archrespite.org/consumer-information.

How Can You Handle the Financial Burden of Dementia?

My dad and I began saving for my mother's care, or perhaps *his* someday, in 2008. Better than nothing, but too late. We wish we had discussed potential financial needs earlier and had imagined some worst-case scenarios and how we would survive them. I've been lucky enough to have resources to help pay a significant portion of the costs of Mom's care. But many people are in a different situation. Every family should become informed about what to do before large bills loom.

An easy-to-read online brochure covers a lot of ground about the basics, including long-term insurance, tax implications, what Medicare does and doesn't cover, and government assistance under the Affordable Health Care act, which ended pre-existing condition exclusions: http://www.alz.org /national/documents/brochure_moneymatters.pdf.

How Can You Keep a Dangerous Driver off the Roads?

One big mistake we made was allowing Mom to continue to drive. We should've heeded Dr. Mesulam's warning and acted on it immediately. Enlisting a physician to tell her she could no longer drive might have lessened the friction within the family. As an option, the internist could have given her a prescription for a driving test at a nearby rehabilitation hospital with the assurance that if she proved she was no threat to herself or others, no one could ground her. She would not have passed.

Advice here concludes that if a stop-driving order from a respected outside authority doesn't work, you may have to disable or remove the car: www.alz.org/care/alzheimers -dementia-and-driving.asp.

An insurance company partnered with MIT's AgeLab on research about dementia and driving. The results include tips for conducting difficult conversations and a one-page agreement for someone with dementia to sign before their judgment becomes clouded: www.thehartford.com/mature -market-excellence/dementia-driving.

What Can Caregivers Do When a Loved One Becomes Incontinent or Aggressive?

These two challenges often drive even the most stoic caregivers, like my dad, to get help or begin a search for long-term care. Online resources focus on what my father had to learn: Show calm even when you're not. Recognize Mom's feelings and respect them. For example, say, "Something spilled on you" instead of "You wet yourself." More here: www.alz.org /care/alzheimers-dementia-incontinence.asp#respond.

For aggression, first rule out pain, then try to find the cause. Music soothes: http://www.alz.org/care/alzheimers -dementia-aggression-anger.asp.

How Can You Find a Good Long-Term-Care Facility While Dodging Thinly Disguised Sales Pitches?

Dad began by calling a company that specialized in placements for people with dementia. He had several long phone talks with an amiable representative in New York. She emailed him a list of local long-term-care options supposedly matching Mom's specific needs—"memory care"—for her disease.

Later, he learned that the company depended on placements. It would've been paid if my father had chosen one of the residences the woman proposed. *Was she really concerned about us?* he wondered. After driving to all of the nearby options, he found Mom's future home on his own.

The visits became a good source of advice for him. Salespeople always accompanied him on tours. Typically, no matter what they said, he knew within a minute whether a facility was right for my mother. But talking to social workers and chief executive officers at each site gave him a fresh perspective on caregiving, in particular with regard to how to tell my mother it was time to move and what he could do to take care of himself and Mom during the transition.

Your tax dollars at work: To connect with service agencies near you, enter your zip code at a US government source, www.eldercare.gov/Eldercare.NET/Public/Index.aspx.

Considering Brain Donation?

An autopsy is the surest way to learn what caused my mom's disease and might also reveal hereditary risks my family might be facing. We agreed to donate her brain to support studies on her condition that could lead to a treatment or cure. But autopsies are expensive, and not every medical center can afford them. Since her case is part of the database where she got her second opinion, researchers there have tracked the course of her disease since 2006. They will pay for the postmortem examination.

Here's a searchable database of brain banks around the world: www.alzforum.org/brain-banks.

Make Sure Your Parents (and You) Each Have a Will

Ensure that your parents and spouse have individual wills. And get one for yourself if you haven't already. The growing number of early-onset dementia cases undercuts the myth that only seniors need wills. To find an attorney near you for wills and other related matters, call the Alzheimer's Association at 800-272-3900.

Assemble Other Essential Documents Now, Whether Someone in Your Family Has Dementia or Not

Around the time of diagnosis, my parents' lawyer also drew up durable powers of attorney for each of them. It was a crucial, low-cost move that allowed my father to pay bills and sign a contract for refinancing their jointly owned home. At the same time, they obtained several other important no-cost documents. Health care proxies named each other as agents empowered to make medical decisions. In 2008, as her own signature began disintegrating toward illegibility, Mom signed a living will, a one-page statement that spelled out her refusal of any "heroic measures." Later Dad, as Mom's agent, used a New York State MOLST (Medical Orders for Life-Sustaining Treatment) to give similar but more detailed instructions to the staff on her floor and anyone who took care of her.

What was missing from this file of formal, boilerplate documents was a personal note from my mother in her own words after she knew she had dementia. That document would have told us more about what she meant. It would have shared her wishes about living and fears about dying—or living with "extreme physical or mental disability." I'm working on my note now:

> *If I ever become irreversibly cognitively impaired, I want my family and loved ones to know that they have my permission and encouragement to move me out of my home into an assisted-living facility if they feel threatened by me, physically or emotionally. If I have a terminal condition, they have my permission to give medicine for comfort measures only, and I accept the decisions they will make on my behalf. They should know that I want them to move on with*

their lives, to be well, and to thrive. I would like them to let go of guilt and to visit me when they can. I want them to witness the reality of whatever condition I am in, but to remember that I believe things aren't always as they seem. I want them to seek joy, to look for angels and God winks, to love each other, and to celebrate life, no matter what form it takes.

ACKNOWLEDGMENTS

want to thank my family for giving me their blessing to tell my version of this story, which affected all of us in different ways. This book would not have been possible without their support. My father read every word of this manuscript for me again and again, offering insights, dates, diaries, and often better phrasing and grammar. His influence is on every page, especially in the Resources section. I loved working on this with you, Dad. Thank you to my brother, Jay, and sister, Ash, for listening, for reading, and for filling in details on memories I'd forgotten. You are my best friends, my heroes, and I don't know what I would do without you. My wonderful in-laws, Doug and Sandy, thank you for always being there (and for being such fun grandparents so I didn't feel as guilty going off to work). Aunt Diana, thank you for all the specifics about our family history, and for reading the manuscript for me to make sure I was getting them right. You are one of the strongest women I know. Thank you to Nancy, for poring over the material, and cheering me on with laughter and tears, in spite of being in a tricky position. Thanks to Dawn, Becky, and Meghan, other hard-working members of my support team at home who helped pick up the pieces so I could write.

Thank you to Mom's tireless caregivers over the years, who have often given solace to my father as well, especially, Laura, Millie, Tsahi, Jacob, Susie, Joanne, Herma, Mary Ann, Maria, Celina, Carissa and Greg. You have a challenging job, and you do it with patience, humor, grace, and kindness.

Thank you to our devoted lifelong family friends: Anna and Bruce, Sheelah and Bill, Jim and Betsy, Larry and Betsy. You all stepped in at crucial times, and this is your story, too. Thanks to Liz and Bill, Karen and Kelley, Robin, Ann, Terri, and Heather for your encouragement and kindness. Thank you to my amazing girlfriends, who listened and asked great questions and helped me figure out what I wanted to say over long, lingering dinners: Tracie, Sheryl, Connie, Cassidy, Nic, Jessi, Missy, Susan, Emily. I adore you. Karen Weingard, you have helped me in more ways than I can count over the years, and given me such insight. Big love and gratitude to you.

Thank you to Michael, for writing the perfect foreword. I admire and appreciate you so much. Thank you to all of the people who took time to talk to me about working with my mom: Tricia Park, Katie Hite, Laura Goodwin, Sue Matthews; and Veronique Enos, Todd Sherer, Holly Teich-holt, and Debi Brooks at the Michael J. Fox Foundation. Your stories added depth and color, and helped me to see Mom in a new light. Thank you to the doctors who helped with medical information: Laurel Coleman, M.D., Eileen H. Bigio, M.D., and Mary S. Mittelmann, D.PH. Thank you to the Alzheimer's Association for being a fantastic resource, especially to Ruth Kolb Drew, Mary Ann Urbasich, Kate Meyer, and Angela Geiger. Thank you to Sarah Smith and *Redbook* for helping me get my message out into the world for the first time, and to Jill Herzig for suggesting I go fur-ther with a book.

Thank you to Mary Ellen, Wade, Amy, Meghan, Sandy, and Susan for being brave early readers of the manuscript. Your insights, helpful criticism, and encouragement helped shape this book and kept me going. Thanks to Chris, Barry, Liz, and J. Karen for sharing your experiences. Thanks Sampson Brueher, for helping me through my computer woes. Bill Simmons and Kendal Marcy, thanks for always answering my texts and emails.

Thank you to Michelle Bega for championing every part of this project, from weighing in on the manuscript to helping me get permissions. You are a treasure. Thank you Anna Holbrook, John Shannon, Lara Porzak, Ben Enos, Jim Shea, and Mandy Johnson for capturing beautiful moments in time with your cameras. And to Sandy Lawrence, Leonard Cohen, Kelley Lovelace, and Brad Paisley for your lovely lyrics.

Thanks to everyone at Link Entertainment, especially Brian Wilkins and Ryan Bundra, for following through and actually making this happen. And to Katherine Latshaw at Folio Literary Management, who offered honesty and encouragement and taught me about the complexities of publishing. Thank you to Joyce Deprest and Harley Neuman, for always having my back.

Many thanks to my fantastic team at Penguin Random House: Molly Stern, Annsley Rosner, Tricia Boczkowski, Jenni Zellner, Tammy Blake, Ellen Folan, Julie Cepler, Gianna Antolos, Courtney Snyder, Cindy Berman, Anna Thompson, and Christopher Brand. Special thanks to my excellent editor, Amanda Patten, who patiently walked me through this process and who imparted wise and insightful suggestions.

Last, thanks to Brad, Huck, and Jasper for your encouragement, enthusiasm, patience, and humor. I love you three guys like crazy. You are one big God wink. And you are where the light especially gets in.

—*KWP*

Photo Credits

P. 6: Lara Porzak; p. 10: Lara Porzak; p. 38: ©1991 Touchstone Pictures; p. 219: Mandy Johnson; p. 244: Anna Holbrook.

All other photos courtesy of the author.

Song Credits

Grateful acknowledgment is made to the following:

Sandra Lawrence: Lyrics from "When I'm Gone" by Sandra Lawrence. All rights reserved. Used by permission of Sandra Lawrence.

Sony/ATV Music Publishing LLC: Lyrics from "Anthem" by Leonard Cohen, copyright © 1992 by Sony/ATV Music Publishing LLC. All rights administered by Sony/ATV Music Publishing LLC, 424 Church Street, Suite 1200, Nash-